The Night Is Normal

. . .

THE
NIGHT
IS
NORMAL

A GUIDE THROUGH SPIRITUAL PAIN

ALICIA BRITT CHOLE

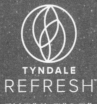

TYNDALE
REFRESH™

Think Well. Live Well. Be Well.

Visit Tyndale online at tyndale.com.

Visit the author online at https://aliciachole.com.

Tyndale, Tyndale's quill logo, *Tyndale Refresh*, and the Tyndale Refresh logo are registered trademarks of Tyndale House Ministries. Tyndale Refresh is a nonfiction imprint of Tyndale House Publishers, Carol Stream, Illinois.

The Night Is Normal: A Guide through Spiritual Pain

For information about special discounts for bulk purchases, please contact Tyndale House Publishers at csresponse@tyndale.com, or call 1-855-277-9400.

Library of Congress Cataloging-in-Publication Data

A catalog record for this book is available from the Library of Congress.

ISBN 978-1-4964-6515-3

Printed in the United States of America

29	28	27	26	25	24	23
7	6	5	4	3		

DEDICATED TO MY BELOVED DAUGHTER, KEONA

Keona, when you were born, I never could have imagined that before your twentieth birthday, you would be well acquainted with life-altering accidents, long-term illnesses, near and dear special needs, irreplaceable losses, and a global pandemic. But I did know this: As you worshiped and followed Jesus, you would lead your generation out of deserts. Over the years, you have allowed the night to season you into a deep and integrous soul. I could not be prouder of the woman you have become, and you have mentored me in more ways than you know.

One of my favorite Keona-mentoring moments occurred when you were only ten. A few weeks after my first occurrence of cancer, you handed me a card with a horse on the outside and the following words etched in bright-pink pen on the inside:

> Dear Mommy, read this card and remember He is always with you and He always loves you. Remember that your family loves you on good days and bad days, on easy days, on hard days. There are always two families who love you, and they are the family of God and us. We will love you if you only need supplements to if you need chemo. We love you no matter what. (Read this card every day.) Your BFF, Keona

I still keep your card near me. And wherever the future carries you, may its truth remain near you: Always remember, my Keo, that you are profoundly loved . . . in every day and through every night.

Contents

PART THREE Disillusionment with Self

PART FOUR Disillusionment with Others

PART ONE

• • •

Navigating
the Night

Chapter 1

. . .

FACING THE STORM
TOGETHER

Perhaps it began on the front porch. Or rather, on the front porches. My family moved every year to a new city, new house, and new school as my dad pursued a new dream. Growing up, the happy constant was the love of my parents and a few traditions like this one.

"Porch" might be a bit generous, though. Often, it was more of a covered doorstep. Big or small, it was a haven for me. Dad worked all day and most weekends, so this was a night tradition. To this day, it remains one of my sweetest memories.

Every once in a while, we started early if we happened to notice the lightning. But most times the tradition began when we heard thunder in the distance. Dad's eyes would brighten as he announced, "A storm is coming!"

When I was little, Dad would scoop me up in his arms and carry me. As I grew too big for scooping, he would hold my hand as we hurried to take our positions on the porch. Then, facing the storm in the darkness, Dad would tuck me under his arm as we sat together in silence (except, of course, when counting seconds between lightning flashes and crackling rumbles).

Sometimes, depending on how porchy the porch was, we stayed outside for the entire storm. But always, we would stay as long as we could, enjoying the wind, rain, "thunderboomers,"[1] and light show together.

Dad decided early on that I would not inherit the family fear of storms. He succeeded. Since I was small, I have associated storms with an invitation to spend time in the safe arms of my dad.

That association eventually—but not immediately—transferred from my earthly dad to my heavenly One. My earliest years as a follower of Jesus were filled with little night and lots of daylight. The first night-storm in my faith actually took me by surprise, and I initially interpreted it as a faith failure instead of an invitation to enrich my relationship with God. Since God mercifully reestablished that connection, the night has hosted my greatest spiritual growth spurts and become a faith-strengthening focus of my studies.

In that sense, I began writing this book a long time ago on a little porch in the middle of the night through the realization that storms are survivable when we view them as relational. The night is filled with holy invitations to grow our love for God.

A disconnect between the night and *growth, nearness, and love* has spiritually shipwrecked many souls. Misinterpreting the night and overwhelmed by spiritual pain, we cut anchor and lose, or abandon, our confidence in God, in our ability to follow God, or in the community of God's people.

This may be where you are right now: adrift, aware of an undercurrent pulling you away from shore into a dark, turbulent sea. It can be frightening when your faith feels ungrounded, untethered, unkept. It certainly has been distressing for me.

You and I may be meeting for the very first time in these pages, but from the beginning, please know that you are not alone. And you are not as far away from home as you may think or as it may feel.

The night is not your enemy.

My goal in this offering is to help you reclaim the night and reinterpret the pain by building (or rebuilding) a framework for spiritual disillusionment.

Thankfully, I did not have to start from scratch. Many brilliant voices and profound pens have gone before me. My small, but hopefully meaningful, contribution is the offering of a visual framework and a set of practical tools for navigating the night.

Part One of this book is foundational. In this first set of chapters, we will wrap our minds around *the concept of spiritual pain and discover how disillusionment is an invitation to love.* Subsequent parts will offer tools for navigating *disillusionment with God* (Part Two), *disillusionment with ourselves* (Part Three), and *disillusionment with God's people* (Part Four). Because even though the night is normal, a lack of tools can make it longer and thicker than it needs to be.

However, if your night seems overwhelming, it is okay to skip ahead to a part that meets a felt need. But please remember to circle back and read Part One. That foundation is our compass through spiritual pain. Knowing where you are headed will make the tools offered here far more effective.

The supplemental materials—appendices, endnotes, and bibliography—contain some of the overflow of my thirty years of study on the subject. To keep the book accessible, I have chosen to present that material as optional but highly recommended reading.

As you begin this journey, I encourage you to bring any uncertainty, frustration, and pain with you. Denial—however polite or well-intended—has no regenerative power. Personally, I honor honest questions (especially thorny ones) as welcome friends, in part because I view their primary purpose as strengthening relationships instead of acquiring answers. It was an early ease with questioning that led me to a lifelong love of learning. And the subject of disillusionment has been my primary study focus since the park-bench crisis you will soon read about.

It might be helpful for you to know two more things about me from the start. First, though I do a bit of writing and speaking, my core calling has always been as a mentor, which means I have had the privilege of wading through a lot of spiritual pain with a lot of stunning hearts and minds.

Second, I am *deeply* concerned about the frailty of our collective faith. God has not changed. But our understanding of what it means to follow Him has undergone an alarming mutation from the dual toxins of mistaking emotions for devotion and viewing abundance as proof of obedience.

Lacking a framework for valuing and processing disillusionment, we assume that spiritual growth prefers the happy day and shuns the not-so-happy night. Consequently, we avoid the night, viewing it as spiritual-formation misfire or a senseless waste of time and potential.

This error is certainly not new, as even a brief reading of the counsel of Job's friends can confirm. But in any age, when an error is elevated to the status of belief, creed, or doctrine, its power to undermine faith is amplified. Untruth can never heal. And truth—not optimism or daylight—is what genuine spiritual growth craves.

Denying the night's place in our faith silences one of faith's wisest teachers and creates an unsustainable version of what it means to follow Jesus.

So, if truth is looking a little fuzzy,

Or hope is sounding more than a little hollow.

If you are trying in vain to silence the questions,

Or find yourself each day just going through the motions.

If it feels like your faith is barely holding itself together,

Or if you have not felt anything in what seems like forever.

If you love God but are unsure if you still like Him,

Or are growing weary of those people who hang out with Him.

If your faith walk has been . . . well, underwhelming,

Or if abandoning ship is becoming an increasingly enticing drawing

If you have often wondered *why* in the midst of the storm,

Or have searched for a way through the pain when daylight is no longer your norm,

Please do not bail yet.

Join me in hope as we explore the gain in spiritual pain. Risk reclaiming the night and reframing disillusionment as an unexpected friend. Your night will not last forever, but within it, there is priceless treasure that is too weighty to be held by sunshine.

I encourage you to resist the urge to outrun or outgun the pain by moving faster, singing louder, or working harder to stuff your soul with distractions. As you may have experienced, such efforts provide only temporary relief until real life reminds us that something else is off-center, that something at our very core is misaligned.

Though spiritual disillusionment can be profoundly unsettling and though pain's terrain can be rocky and rough, the path toward a healthier, hope-filled view of the night is not unknown. A "great cloud of witnesses" (Hebrews 12:1) has gone before us. Our generation has simply lost the way in our shared illusion that faith always needs full sun to flourish.

No, the night is normal.

In fact, the night is necessary.

Personally, the night is among my faith's oldest and most generous of mentors.

Chapter 2

. . .

NIGHT-FAITH

In hindsight, it was unwise to sit alone in that forgotten, unkept park. But sit I did, head in hands, unconsciously rocking, desperately trying to make my faith

stay put,

stay whole,

simply . . . stay.

The picnic bench on which I perched looked like my faith felt: weathered, unstable, and beyond repair. Those driving by might have thought, *That girl needs to be careful! It's not safe for her to be in that park alone.* But physical danger was the least of my worries.

The sun tried to warm me as it rose, but even the hot Texas sun seemed powerless to light up the night within me. Undeterred, the sun then tried to warn me as it set. I appreciated the gesture but lacked the energy to care. Spiritual pain had depleted my reserves.

There was no blood.

There had been no documentable tragedy.

The battle within, however, had been brutal.

I was struggling with the character—with the very nature—of God.

How on earth did I get here? I winced.

Jesus had interrupted my atheistic worldview just a few years earlier, right before I began my freshman year of college. Meeting Him was most certainly not my idea. As far as I was concerned, there was no God to meet. Clearly, God had not created humans; humans had created God in a desperate (but futile) effort to fill gaps and calm fears. I was pro-reality, not anti-religion. And as a realist, I simply preferred unanswered questions over fairy tales. (Enough said.)

But God's people can be quite wearisome. An especially nice one kept asking me to church until I finally said yes just to keep her quiet. Unsuspecting me went from, *There is no God* to *Oh my God!* in about ninety minutes that Sunday morning. I was awestruck by God's existence and love. *This changes everything*, I thought. And it did. I was no longer alone; Jesus was with me. As He said to the first disciples, "I am the light of the world. Whoever follows me will never walk in darkness, but will have the light of life" (John 8:12).

What a relief—darkness is behind me!

(Or so I thought.)

Maybe this is what you thought too? If so, like me, you might have been more than a little confused when the Light of the World began to dispel the darkness in your heart but not the night in your life.

Later on, I would realize that the promise in this verse was not that darkness would everywhere be banished but that God's light would never, ever vanish. John 8:12 is a spiritual echo of a physical reality God established long before any of us ever learned to be afraid of the dark.

> God said, "Let there be lights in the expanse of the sky to separate the day from the night. . . ." God made two great lights—the greater light to govern the day and the lesser light to govern the night. . . . And God saw that it was good.
> GENESIS 1:14, 16, 18

In the beginning, God's night-light ensured that absolute darkness would not utterly eclipse us. He would always leave a light on, day and night. Jesus' words expanded that ancient assurance from outer-space to inner-space: His followers would have the companionship of His light during each day and through every night.

This is important because we tend to think that spiritual growth prefers one over the other. We tend to forget that the night (not just the light) was also God's creation.

> Now the earth was formless and empty, darkness was over the surface of the deep, and the Spirit of God was hovering over the waters. And God said, "Let there be light," and there was light. God saw that the light was good, and he separated the light from the darkness. God called the light "day," and the darkness he called "night." And there was evening, and there was morning— the first day.
> GENESIS 1:2-5

In the Creation story, day complemented (as opposed to voided) the night. It seems that night-faith was as much a part of God's "in the beginning" goodness as day-faith. Pre-sin, pre-fall, pre-curse, and pre-drama, night was one of the original residents of Eden.

By God's design, every day contains (roughly) twenty-four hours, which means that faith in God is to be lived out during both the day and the night. Physically, however, we have a rather long history of efforts to eliminate, or at least shorten, the night. With candles or clicks, every age has tried to make the night bow to its perceived need for more light and less darkness.

Thankfully, we are slowly regaining a respect for the night's healing powers as researchers affirm the clear connection between darkness, sleep, immune system health, and mental and emotional wellness.[1] Even so, we still are reticent to respect the night spiritually. We prefer to grow by day, thank you. We prefer faith in full sun. We prefer to see clearly, to know much, and to walk confidently into a well-lit future.

But what if spiritual nights are also essential? What if avoiding the night is sabotaging the health of our souls? What if there is something we need in the night that cannot be found in the day?

This was definitely part of my struggle on that park bench. I was desperately trying to climb out of the night because I perceived it as failure, especially in contrast to what I had experienced up to that point.

My first steps with Jesus had been flooded by the brightness of day-faith. Throughout college, in between classes, I stared at Jesus in the Scriptures, captivated by His character. God's Word was alive. His presence was tangible. His work of healing was discernible. My newfound freedom was measurable. Those university years were a greenhouse of growth for me because every time I said, "I believe," some smart someone nearby would ask, "Why?" The continuous opposition kept my heart tender and my religion lean. Of course, there were many areas of struggle as I followed Jesus, but even then, I felt carried in full sun.

That day in the park, however, all I felt was pain. For months, I had been thinking myself into exhaustion, trying to wrap my mind around mysteries beyond me. Nothing made sense anymore. It seemed that I had somehow failed my faith, and now my faith was about to fail me.

In hindsight, God was inviting me into night-faith. And though I could never have anticipated it, night-faith would soon lead me into something far more satisfying than understanding and far more powerful than peace. All that pain was expanding territory for the last thing I expected and the very thing I was afraid to lose: my love for God.

That journey—from the pain, through the night, into love—is the entire focus of this book. *The Night Is Normal* is a summons to sit at the feet of a forgotten mentor: spiritual disillusionment.

In the coming chapters, we will dive deeply into the concept of disillusionment, and at the end of the book I will return to the park bench and share the image God used to help me choose to free-fall into love. But first, I will offer a working definition of disillusionment that will be key to the creation of a helpful, hope-filled framework within which you can navigate your nights.

Chapter 3

· · ·

THAT
STARTLING
"POP"

"Excuse me, I think that you made a mistake," I began with polite confidence.

"Where?" queried my even more confident (but frankly, less polite) English professor.

"Here, where you took off points and wrote 'NOT A REAL WORD,'" I replied, pointing to the obvious on my essay.

"But it's not a real word. Have you looked it up?" the professor said with a smirk.

"Well, no, but everyone knows what it means: it's common knowledge," I said aghast.

Crickets.

"Huh. Well, if you find it in a dictionary, be sure to let me know," the professor concluded, showing me the door.

Challenge accepted, I marched myself straight to the nearest campus library. One hour later, after scouring every dictionary available, I walked back to my dorm in a daze and called my dad.

"Dad, *coveryou* isn't in the dictionary. How could it have completely escaped the notice of Merriam-Webster and all of Oxford? My professor marked my essay down because he said it's not a real word."

I could almost hear Dad's warm smile over the phone.

"Well, Daughter," he offered, "it's a real word *to us.* . . ."

It is true. All the way up to and through my first semester of college English, I was absolutely certain that *coveryou* was a spelling bee–certified, universally valid and valuable member of the English language. We used the term daily in our home. At bedtime, Mom or Dad would hold up a blanket and ask, "Cover you?" Nodding my yes, I would snuggle happily under yet another layer of love. My assumption that everyone knew and understood the term was so uncontested, I never even looked *coveryou* up. Which speaks to my certainty, because I was *always* looking words up.

When I was a child, my parents would find me up past my bedtime, hidden in a closet with a flashlight sneaking in a few more minutes to read . . . the dictionary. Words—their origin stories and modern textures— have always fascinated me. The particular word we are about to study has intrigued me for decades.

Still, why devote precious space to the establishment of a definition? Why take the time—specifically, three entire chapters—to trace a word's origin story?

Because meaning matters and misunderstandings can be costly. In real life, the fallout of assumptions about the meaning of words can range from humorous to disastrous. In college, *coveryou* only cost me a few precious grade points and some mild (to moderate) embarrassment. But in history, wars have been waged over words.

To the point for our context, faith has been discarded over this word.

For many, if not most, *disillusionment* sounds (and feels) dark and doomy. It is a term we only call upon to communicate profound and seemingly permanent loss, such as the loss of innocence, trust, or hope. Since the word appears thoroughly negative, we assume that the experience is equally negative and, understandably, avoid disillusionment in all realms, inclusive of our spiritual lives.

This assumption, however, can be far more dangerous than we might imagine. Why? Because disillusionment is not all loss. When we are disillusioned, loss is making way within us for a powerful gain.

Historically a relatively rare word,[1] *disillusionment* is technically constructed from the prefix *dis-*, the noun *illusion*, and the suffix *-ment*, as follows according to the *Oxford English Dictionary*:

dis-	Latin prefix implying reversal, aversion, removal, or negation.[2]
illusion[3]	A mental state involving the attribution of reality to what is unreal; a false conception or idea; a deception, delusion, fancy.[4]
-ment	From Latin *–mentum*; a suffix forming nouns from verbs (to denote the result or product of the action of the verb).[5]

The word describes the act (*-ment*) of removing or negating (*-dis*) false ideas (*illusions*).[6] Whereas removing an illusion about Santa Claus might be troublesome, removing an illusion about God, our faith in God, or the people of God can rattle us to the core. Spiritual disillusionment occurs when reality challenges our expectations about life in God. It is a form of soul-sorrow in which we think,

Wait a minute.

I thought that God would . . .

I thought that as a believer I could . . .

I thought that God's people should . . .

The good news is that such sorrow holds within it the unexpected gift of a more accurate tomorrow. Because disillusionment is not all loss. Losing an illusion opens the way to gaining a reality. Removing false ideas clears a path to finding truer ideas. The soul-deep sadness of disillusionment challenges and then refines and purifies our beliefs with the fire of Truth.

Which is why my personal definition of disillusionment is *the painful gaining of reality.*

Without question, the process is less than pleasant. But we dare not mistake unpleasant for unfruitful. For example, when it dawns on us that obedience to God can lead us straight into deserts, is that more like Jesus or less like Jesus? When our humanity humbles us, increasing our gratitude for grace, is that a step forward or a step backward in maturity? When we discover that, even in the Church, privileges and influence do not always correlate with purity and integrity, is that a sign of wisdom or foolishness?

No doubt, the stories behind such realizations are dripping with pain. But the disillusionment resulting from those stories contains promise. The loss of illusions is a positive thing; it is evidence that we are *growing.*

Though startling, the process is actually a gift. It reminds us that living faith can never be reduced to lifeless formulas. Formulas gut faith of relationship. And if faith is anything, it is relational.

The Christian faith is a duet to be lived out *with God,* not alone in our heads. Our faith is *in God,* not in our own understanding.

Though needed and noble, our efforts to study and explain God (i.e., theology) can never completely contain God. As we follow Jesus, it is natural for us to collect assumptions about how we think life in God should play out. And it is a gift to us when reality kindly corrects those assumptions through disillusionment. After all, one of the Holy Spirit's primary jobs is to "guide [us] into all truth" (John 16:13). Which means that, as we walk with God, there is always more truth ahead of us than behind us.

Oswald Chambers addressed this hidden gain in disillusionment while writing about World War I:

> During the war many a man has come to find the difference between his creed and God. At first a man imagines he has backslidden because he has lost belief in his beliefs, but later on he finds he has gained God, that is, he has come across reality. . . .

> It does not follow because a man has lost belief in his beliefs that therefore he has lost faith in God. Many a man has been led to the frontiers of despair by being told he has backslidden, whereas what he has gone through has revealed that his belief in his beliefs is not God. Men have found God by going through hell, and it is the ones who have been face to face with these things who can understand what Job went through.[7]

Job's disillusionment is legendary. In the night, pain strained and sifted his beliefs. Day-faith had taken Job far, but night-faith is what ushered him (and what can usher us) into new dimensions of devotion to God.

Like a balloon too small for how much air it needs to hold, our assumptions about who God is and what it means to follow Him often pop from the pressure of the finite (us) trying to contain and explain the Infinite (Him).

All of which reminds me of that fabulous interaction in C. S. Lewis's Chronicles of Narnia when Lucy says to Aslan, "You're bigger," and Aslan responds, "Every year you grow, you will find me bigger."[8]

Evidently, a healthy faith will pop a lot of balloons in its lifetime. As we are schooled by reality, we see God more accurately. The challenge is to reframe that startling pop and begin to associate it with a celebration instead of a funeral.

> *POP.*
>
> *Oh wow, there goes another assumption.*
>
> *I guess God is even bigger than I thought He was.*
>
> *Evidently, I'm growing!*

So we continue to study God (theology) and life keeps reminding us that our greatest thoughts are still too small (POP) and with each cycle through disillusionment, our capacity to love God (for who He really is) expands.

This is why I believe that disillusionment is an unexpected friend of spiritual formation.[9] However painful the loss of illusions may be, reality is a friend of intimacy with God. Because, as Dan B. Allender and Tremper Longman III have stated, "reality is where we meet God."[10]

God is profoundly present to you, right here, right now. He is the ultimate realist. Losing illusions and gaining reality frees you to be more fully present to Him.

So, if you are disillusioned, be encouraged: honest living often leads to the humble leaving of happy but unhelpful illusions.

Chapter 4

. . .

WHAT'S IN A WORD, PART ONE

This would be the perfect moment for a robust biblical word study on disillusionment. However, the word does not make even one appearance in my study Bible. In fact, in a search of over forty English Bible translations, *disillusion*, *disillusioned*, and *disillusionment* were entirely absent in the New Testament and made only seven appearances (scattered throughout four older translations) in the Old Testament canon.[1]

As a theological term, *disillusionment* is missing in the Bible. The word simply escapes us. The experience, however, does not. In Scripture, as in literature, we tend to *feel* disillusionment more than *name* it. We communicate the painful gaining of reality through tales and tears more than letters and labels.

Tracing that communication has been a fascinating venture for me![2] Some of that research can be found in the table which runs parallel to my thoughts in this chapter. Though you are most welcome to skim—or even skip—it, the student in me simply cannot omit it. Additionally, appendix D contains a commentary on this table if you would like to dive a little deeper into the terms.

1500 YEARS OF TERMS USED TO CAPTURE THE CONCEPT OF SPIRITUAL PAIN

Name, Era, Profession	Term: Example and/or Definition
Pseudo-Dionysius (6th Century), theologian, philosopher	*A Ray of Darkness:*[3] "Unto this Darkness which is beyond all Light we pray that we may come, and may attain unto vision through the loss of sight and knowledge, and that in ceasing thus to see or to know we may learn to know that which is beyond all perception and understanding (for this emptying of our faculties is true sight and knowledge)."[4]
Anonymous author of *The Cloud of Unknowing* (14th Century), monk	*Darkness, a cloud of unknowing:* "a lacking of knowing; as all that thing that thou knowest not, or else that thou hast forgotten, it is dark to thee."[5]
John of the Cross (1542–1591), priest, saint	*La Noche Oscura (The Dark Night):* Consisting of the *Passive Night of the Senses* and the *Passive Night of the Spirit*, the *Dark Night* is a soul's pilgrimage toward oneness with God. "[T]his dark night of contemplation should first of all annihilate and undo [the soul] in its meannesses, bringing it into darkness, aridity, affliction and emptiness; for the light which is to be given to it is a Divine light of the highest kind, which transcends all natural light, and which by nature can find no place in the understanding."[6]
Georg Wilhelm Friedrich Hegel (1770–1831), philosopher	*Unhappy Consciousness (unglückliches Bewußtsein)* or *Soul of Despair:* "the 'grief and longing' of the self which yearns for unity ('aims to be absolute') but experiences only inner division at every turn."[7] "the disunity of the *self* before God."[8]
Søren Kierkegaard (1813–1855), philosopher, theologian, poet	*Sickness unto Death* or *Despair:* "Despair is a sickness in the spirit, in the self."[9] "The despairing man cannot die; no more than 'the dagger can slay thoughts' can despair consume the eternal thing, the self, which is the ground of despair, whose worm dieth not, and whose fire is not quenched."[10] "[D]espair is the 'agonizing contradiction' internal to the self in which the basic elements of selfhood stand in fundamental 'disrelationship.'"[11] "not merely as incompleteness of the self, but as incompleteness *before God*, as sin . . . a 'Christian discovery . . . only the Christian knows what is meant by the sickness unto death.'"[12]
C. H. Spurgeon (1834–1892), preacher, pastor	*Agony of Soul:*[13] despair, the "doubting [of] God's gracious character and the promises of his word."[14]
Sigmund Freud (1856–1939), neurologist, founding father of psychoanalysis	*Mourning:* "the reaction to the loss of a loved person, or to the loss of some abstraction which has taken the place of one, such as one's country, liberty, an ideal and so on."[15] "Mourning as Freud conceived it was essentially conservative, only consolidating, repairing, and rescuing lost parts of the ego from the wreckage inflicted upon it by the commands of reality."[16]

Clearly, thoughtful souls have been writing about spiritual pain for a long, long time. Over the centuries, in their shared quest to wrap words around the night, some authors have coined poetic phrases like *ray of darkness*, *cloud of unknowing*, and *the absence that sanctifies*, while others have called upon more common words such as *despair*, *agony*, and *mourning*.

So, why focus on disillusionment above so many other available options? Why not choose something simpler and more accessible, like *grief, suffering, angst, disappointment, agony*, or *crisis*?[17]

While it is true that all these expressions overlap in giving voice to soul-sorrow, by very definition, there is an element in disillusionment that is unique. As we discovered in the previous chapter, disillusionment is one of the rare terms that guarantees gain in the midst of loss. As such, it is related to (but not a certain synonym for) other, more modern expressions. For example:

> Though disillusionment is no stranger to *grief* or *suffering*, those who grieve and suffer are not always disillusioned.
>
> Though often expressed by emotions like *angst* or *disappointment*, disillusionment is not exclusively sourced in emotions but rather in the mysterious connection between mind and spirit.
>
> Though the experience of disillusionment can be marked by *agony*, disillusionment can also be numbing.
>
> Though sometimes preceded by a *crisis*, disillusionment can equally occur in the absence of a crisis.[18]

All these words communicate powerful feelings and states, yet disillusionment is still *other*. That otherness is the very key that casts *hope* as a lead character in our journeys through the night.

Hope is really what my dad gave me on the front porch through many years of storms. His calm presence reframed what could have been only

Name, Era, Profession	Term: Example and/or Definition
Max Weber (1864–1920), sociologist, historian, philosopher, economist, one of the founders of sociology	*Disenchantment:* the decline in Western culture in beliefs in magic.[19]
Melanie Klein (1882–1960), psychoanalyst, coined the term *reparation*	*Pining:* mourning, originating in early mother-infant relationship and resurfacing periodically in adulthood.[20]
C. S. Lewis (1898–1963), scholar, novelist, apologist	*Iconoclasm:* the shattering of God-ideas by God Himself.[21]
Béla Vassady (1902–1992), theologian, historian	*Despair:* "For there are two kinds of despair or sorrow. The first one St. Paul calls the 'sorrow of the world' which sweeps man into the turbulent waters of disillusionment, lethargy, desire for death, and suicide, and thus inevitably 'worketh death.' The other kind of despair St. Paul calls 'godly sorrow' which prepares the soil for the outlook involved in the statement, 'Whom the Lord loveth, he reproveth.' From this soil springs that 'repentance unto salvation' which branches out into a new hope and a new obedience."[22]
Julian Norris Hartt (1911–2010), theologian	*Despair* (as a theological motivation): "a feeling or sense of hopelessness. . . . A person in despair may be doing a great deal, but all that he does is under a sentence of hopelessness."[23]
Heinz Kohut (1913–1981), psychoanalyst, developed self-psychology	*De-idealization:* as described by Homans, "refers to the pre-oedipal line of development, the figure of the mother more than that of the father, and to issues of unconscious self-esteem, merger, self-cohesion, grandiosity, and the loss of ideals."[24]
Thomas Merton (1915–1968), Trappist monk	*The Absence that Sanctifies:* when God "is present and His presence is affirmed and adored by the absence of everything else. . . . In the absence that sanctifies, God empties the soul of every image that might become an idol and of every concern that might stand between our face and His."[25]
Peter Homans (1930–2009), psychologist, professor	*De-idealization:* "an inner psychological sequence of states, characteristic of adult life, with a beginning, middle, and end. It is developmentally grounded"[26] and "an essential component in normal development, and, like melancholia, it includes emptiness in the inner world, as well as a sense of loss in the external environment. . . . [D]e-idealization is progressive in its outcome, leading as it does to new values and new psychological structure."[27]
David R. Blumenthal (1938–), rabbi, professor of Judaic studies at Emory University	*Theological Despair:* "a distrust of the holiness of our history, a doubting of the One Who lends meaning to that history."[28] "Despair is more profound than doubt. It runs much deeper than distress. Despair is a questioning of the very frame of meaning in our lives."[29]

frightening into something that was always enlightening. Yes, the night was dark and I could not see my way through it. But, facing the darkness together, I realized that no storm lasted forever. And more importantly, I discovered that every storm strengthened our relationship.

This is the hope that I pray is rising within you as we reframe disillusionment together. Your nights, though normal, are not eternal. And within each one is an invitation to strengthen your relationship with God.

1500 YEARS OF TERMS USED TO CAPTURE
THE CONCEPT OF SPIRITUAL PAIN (CONTINUED)

Name, Era, Profession	Term: Example and/or Definition
Gerald G. May (1940–2005), psychiatrist, psychologist, theologian	*The Dark Night:* "The dark night is a profoundly good thing. It is an ongoing spiritual process in which we are liberated from attachments and compulsions and empowered to live and love more freely."[30]
Jerome T. Walsh (1942–2021), professor of theology and biblical studies	*Qoheleth:* used by Walsh to represent one who, like Qoheleth, the writer of Ecclesiastes, sincerely arrives at an isolating conclusion that God is "arbitrary" or "undecipherable." God is the "personal, willful power behind all of life's unfairness."[31]
James S. Reitman (1949–), theologian	*Disillusionment:* "when our deeply held aspirations or expectations are decisively frustrated. . . . such disillusionment may well reflect an existential angst that in the end God will remain silent and/or absent."[32]
Philip Yancey (1949–), author	*Disappointment:* "when the actual experience of something falls far short of what we anticipate."[33] *The Pain of Betrayal:* "The pain of a lover who wakes up and suddenly realizes *it's all over.* He had staked his life on God, and God had let him down."[34]
Gene Edward Veith Jr. (1951–), provost, professor of literature	*Disillusionment:* the unfortunate and potentially faith-shattering experience of those who have not understood that we are all sinners and that, because of sin, "offenses will indeed come."[35]
Daniel Berthold-Bond (1953–), professor of philosophy	*Despair:* "the inability to reconcile opposites internal to the self."[36]
Rabbi Elie Kaplan Spitz (1954–), rabbi, professor of philosophy	*Despair:* a "deep and dark, heavy and desperate" experience that "comes from the cumulative weight of burdens—losses, wounds, responsibilities, and questions of purpose."[37]
John H. Coe (1956–), professor of philosophy and spiritual theology	*Dark Night of the Soul:* times "in which the Spirit secretly does a deep work in the human spirit—a work that is so profound but feels so foreign to the Christian's experience that it is often interpreted as the absence of God."[38]
Simon D. Podmore (1977–), professor of systematic theology	*Despair:* an experience through which "the self . . . can die to itself and be reborn through faith in the blessed impossibility of the resurrection of the dead God."[39]

Chapter 5

. . .

WHAT'S IN A WORD,
PART TWO

To keep hope central in the nights of our faith, we need to distinguish disillusionment from three terms that are often used as near (and negative) synonyms: *cynicism*, *skepticism*, and *despair*.

Early *cynicism* was a complex and controversial fifth-century Greek school of thought in which cynics lived unattached to material things and indifferent (and in protest) to societal norms. Today, a cynic is "a person disposed to rail or find fault; one who shows a disposition to disbelieve in the sincerity or goodness of human motives and actions; a sneering fault-finder."[1]

In other words, nothing and no one is ever *good enough*.

The meal lacked this.

The movie needed that.

The party could have been better.

The day should have been brighter.

The job pays the bills but isn't satisfying.

The friendship helps the loneliness but isn't exciting.

Though often excused with "I'm just being honest," it seems to me that cynicism is more about interior discontent than honesty. Honesty is a means of honoring reality, whereas cynicism is a focus on any negative at the expense of all positive.

Surely all of us have at least one friend or loved one who leans cynic— who sees even full cups as empty and seems to instinctively do the very opposite of finding the proverbial silver lining. Our wired age is fertile soil for the proliferation of cynicism. Hidden safely behind screens, our generation can find fault effortlessly and anonymously.

Personally, I find chronic cynicism exhausting. The combination of inaccuracy and never-enoughness wears on me. Yet disillusionment does something different in my soul. Temporary sadness over whatever illusion I have lost gives way to a quiet gratitude for what always remains.

Over a century ago, Oswald Chambers contrasted cynicism with disillusionment in the classic *My Utmost for His Highest*: "Disillusionment means that there are no more false judgments in life . . . the disillusionment which comes from God brings us to the place where we see men and women as they really are, and yet there is no cynicism, we have no stinging, bitter things to say."[2]

In this comparison, Chambers hints at the hope in disillusionment. Whereas cynicism is a bitter lens, disillusionment is an open door through which we lose "false judgments" and gain accuracy. Uninfected realism is one of disillusionment's potential outcomes.

Whereas a cynic knows no good, a skeptic knows nothing with certainty.

Early *skepticism*[3] was a second- and third-century Greek and Indian movement that elevated inquiry, suspended certainty, and sometimes manifested in a professional disbelief in belief. Today, a skeptic is one who "doubts the possibility of real knowledge of any kind; one who holds that there are no adequate grounds for certainty as to the truth of any proposition whatsoever."[4]

I first encountered this line of thinking in a college philosophy class. From day one, the professor laid out his thesis that nothing can be known with certainty. Then, for weeks, he brought in various optical illusions and experiments designed to erode confidence in our ability to perceive anything with accuracy. A lens in a jar warped our line of sight so we reached for an object in vain. A sound bounced off a wall, and we guessed its source in error. He then leapt from the unreliability of our senses to the unreliability of history and finally to the unreliability of religious beliefs. (As a humorous sidenote, for our final we had to take a belief that people were certain of and show how, at best, it was a mere guess. I wrote my paper on atheism.)

Though an entertaining class and despite the obvious contradiction (how can anyone be certain that nothing is certain?), my lasting takeaway was the glaring unsustainability of philosophical skepticism. Whereas disillusionment leads me further into reality, skepticism places reality further and further out of reach.

Ivan Sergeevich Turgenev contrasted disillusionment with skepticism in an 1859 novel entitled *A Nest of Gentry*.[5] The following excerpt is a conversation between two of the main characters in which the first, Mikhavelich, is describing his recent spiritual journey:

> "I've changed in many ways . . . although I haven't changed in the important, essential ways. I still believe in goodness and truth. But I don't merely believe in them, now I have faith—yes, I have faith, I have faith. . . . Let me read my most recent poem aloud to you—I've expressed my deepest convictions in it. . . ."

> Mikhavelich began to read his poem. It was rather long, and ended with the following lines:

> *I gave myself over to new feelings with all my heart,*

My soul became childlike.

And I've burned everything I once worshiped,

And now worship everything I once burned.

Laveretskii listened to him at length . . . and a spirit of antagonism arose within him. . . . [A] heated argument had broken out between them, one of those endless arguments only Russians engage in. . . .

"What are you then, after all this? Disillusioned?" Mikhavelich demanded to know at one o'clock in the morning. . . . "Well, if you aren't disillusioned, you're a *skepteek*, which is even worse."[6]

The spiritual pain captured in the words "I've now burned everything I once worshiped," transcends time and culture. Such a phrase describes an agonizing loss of illusions. Yet, as painful as it was, disillusionment was still preferred over skepticism. Why? Why did the author describe skepticism as "worse"?

In its most benign form, skepticism can simply be intellectual doubt that inspires further study. However, a confirmed skeptic is not simply a doubter but somewhat of a philosophical agnostic; someone who ascribes to the "doctrine that true knowledge or knowledge in a particular area is uncertain."[7]

Surely we live in an age of global skepticism. The question "Who really knows?" now has creed-like weight in our culture. My old professor would be pleased. In our day, the only acceptable thing to be certain of is uncertainty.

Our generation no longer capitalizes *truth*; we keep it small so that we do not offend. And so, we cheer one another on to "find your own [small *t*] truth," unconstrained by history, logic, or even evidence. Because, after all . . . *who really knows?*

Perhaps such skepticism was described as "worse" in the novel because the professional skeptic has no hope. Uncertainty only begets more uncertainty, and loss only leads to more loss. However, for the disillusioned, uncertainty leads to discovery, and loss leads to gain.

Yes, the disillusioned may burn things they used to worship. But, unlike the skeptic, that is not their final end. As ideas and ideals are reduced to ashes, something ancient is reborn—something of the faith, hope, and love exemplified by the earliest followers of Jesus. Then we, too, share in Mikhavelich's celebration: "But I don't merely believe in them, now I have faith—yes, I have faith, I have faith." Such is the power and potential of spiritual disillusionment.

Unlike cynicism and skepticism, *despair* is not a school of thought but rather a state of hopelessness. Psychologically, despair is "the emotion or feeling of hopelessness, that is, that things are profoundly wrong and will not change for the better. Despair is one of the most negative and destructive of human affects."[8] If you, or someone you love, has ever believed that life is not worth living, you understand exactly how devastating the absence of hope can be for the soul.

In this way, disillusionment and despair are more antonyms than synonyms. Whereas disillusionment is a loss of illusions, despair is a loss of hope. This distinction is one of the primary reasons that we desperately need a viable framework for processing spiritual pain.

If we do not normalize the night in the life of faith, we can easily mistake spiritual darkness for spiritual death.[9] Loss then gives way to despair. But countless saints who have gone before us affirm that the loss in the night—the spiritual pain in disillusionment—is meant to give way to love. As Abraham J. Twerski explained,

> The Talmud says that Moses asked God why there is suffering, and God answered that as long as a person inhabits a physical body, he cannot possibly understand this. Following the

revelation at Sinai, the Torah says, "Moses approached the thick cloud where God was."

One might think that God's immanent presence would be in brightness, but Moses knew better. It is in darkness of life that we may find God.[10]

Finding God is the treasure of disillusionment. There, buried in the night, is a purified relationship with Him that can offer satisfaction to the cynic, solid ground to the skeptic, and life-giving hope to those drowning in despair.

Chapter 6

. . .

A RELATIONAL
CYCLE

Has *God* ever not been who you thought He was?

Have *you* ever not been who you hoped you were?

Have *the people of God* ever not been who you needed them to be?

In short, have you ever been disillusioned?

Early on in my faith walk, I did a study chronicling every conflict I could find in the Scriptures from Genesis to Revelation. Nearly every page preserved some form of relational pain laid bare for the ages. The unsanitized nature of the Bible inspired my confidence in its authenticity. (Frankly, something purely man-made would have applied more filters.)

During that study, in story upon story, I began to see and sketch a pattern in spiritual pain. Any illustration is at some level a simplification, and though the following image cannot capture the complexity of spiritual pain, its intent is to illustrate the position and potential of disillusionment in the life of faith.

Our relationships with God, with our own faith, and with people of faith seem to share in common a cycle that often begins with an inspiring and intoxicating substance I will clumsily call *joyful anticipation*.

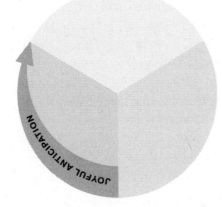

Joy describes a "vivid emotion of pleasure arising from a sense of well-being or satisfaction; the feeling or state of being highly pleased or delighted; exultation of spirit; gladness, delight."[1] *Anticipation* is defined as a feeling of "excitement about something that is going to happen."[2]

Naming this first stage in the cycle of relationships has been a struggle. I have used *infatuation* when speaking and *delight* in my dissertation. But infatuation has, definitionally, an undercurrent of foolishness, and delight does not depict how we tend to assume this glad stage is a deposit on an unknown future. It is difficult to find one word to communicate that initial heartfelt blush, that authentic, happy expectation of continued good. Since one all-encompassing word escapes me, allow me to illustrate these two.

Joyful anticipation is when . . .

> You experience the forgiveness of God, and all is right and new in the world.

> You meet that special someone, and there are stars in your eyes.

You go into business with your best friend because, with Jesus at the center, what could possibly go wrong?

You find a dream mentor who obviously walks on water.

Fresh starts, starry eyes, confident expectation, honest admiration—this is joyful anticipation at its finest. Yes, the source of such anticipation can range from unfounded infatuation to well-researched speculation. But it is important to remember that the joy is real. That warm, promising feeling is a genuine emotion. If there is an illusion in joyful anticipation, it is its permanence. Sooner or later, life will carry us into the next stage in the cycle of relationships, which is *disillusionment*, the painful gaining of reality.

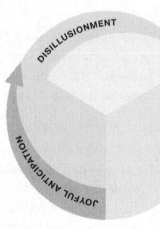

Disillusionment is when . . .

Your faith falls flat.

You are having trouble connecting with that special someone.

Your best friend is neither the best nor a friend.

You have a front-row view of your mentor's humanity.

And, potentially even more devastating, disillusionment is also when . . .

A loved one takes their life.

A miracle pregnancy miscarries.

A beloved leader is tormented by temptation.

A visionary steps out in faith into what seems like failure.

A sincere soul has not sensed God's presence in years.

Disillusionment is when our assumptions about God, our lives as believers, and other God-followers collide with reality. The shock shakes loose illusions. We begin to see more clearly. And God—through the painful gaining of reality—invites us to grow.

We realize that . . .

Emotion is not synonymous with devotion.

Two becoming one is a process.

New circumstances introduce unexpected challenges into established relationships.

And leaders are still learners.

We begin to understand that . . .

Grieving with God is what keeps mystery uninfected.

Life is a gift even when its length makes no sense.

Temptation is not a synonym for sin.

Outcome does not get to retroactively judge obedience.

And faith is not a feeling.

This is disillusionment. This is spiritual pain. And this is a real problem because our culture does not teach us how to live past this point in life, let alone in faith.

We live in an age that mistakenly calls joyful anticipation *love*[3] and, therefore, views spiritual disillusionment as *failure*. So, when *love fails*, our culture counsels us to *bail*.

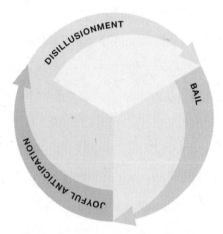

Can you see our generation stuck in this cycle?

Anticipation, disillusionment, bail. Delight, disillusionment, bail. Infatuation, disillusionment, bail.

On the threshold of spiritual growth—on the verge of gaining realities that infuse faith with depth—we interpret the pain as failure and bail. Church after church, community after community, tradition after tradition, even god after god, the cycle starts again as we continue our search for a spiritual life (or even just a life) that lacks pain.

Try, try again.

Or not.

(Many are choosing "or not" these days.)

In the absence of a theological framework within which to recognize the night as normal in our faith, we mistake the night for nothingness. Without certainty that disillusionment is a well-traveled path *within* faith, we assume that experiencing disillusionment somehow means that we have moved outside the faith.

No and no.

The night is normal.

Disillusionment is evidence of growth, not decay. In disillusionment, God invites us to reframe questions as companions, to see that our senses neither create nor negate His presence, and to experience the fellowship of Jesus' suffering.[4] In disillusionment, shiny (yet sometimes shallow) ideals are lost, as deeper (yet initially duller) reality is gained.

So, if you are disillusioned, please, borrow my hope: another path besides "bail" is available to you. A path that will lift you upward instead of pushing you downward. A path that will help you navigate the night with courage.

But before exploring that upward possibility, we must first come to grips with why "bail" has such a pull on us—with why it is so difficult to apply Jesus' "remain in me" (John 15:4) to the night of disillusionment.

Chapter 7

. . .

BETWEEN ILLUSION AND REALITY

"No-man's-land" is a rather ominous term used in reference to uninhabit-able spaces, such as land between foes, dangerous regions, deserted build-ings, or, figuratively, "a state of confusion or uncertainty."[1] Only recently did I learn that it is also an actual place. Nomans Land, Massachusetts, is a real 612-acre island that was used as a bombing range in the twentieth century.

Both as an address and a noun, no-man's-land describes territory that is unlivable. One simply cannot stay there (let alone set up a home there) for long.

In some ways, the space between illusion and reality can feel like a no-man's-land. In between what we thought we knew and what we are begin-ning to understand, the tension can seem uninhabitable. This is one of the reasons it is so tempting to bail right on the brink of insight and growth.

Avoiding illusions altogether may appear to be a smart strategy, but that state is more uninhabitable than any real or allegorical no-man's-land.

We are finite beings in relationship with an infinite Creator living out our days on an earth (not to mention in a universe) too complex to fully comprehend.

No wonder we have illusions!

Most are not innately evil.

If fact, most are not even consciously chosen.

While it is possible to create illusions willfully (as when a child asks, "Is it okay if I believe in Santa a little while longer?") or to suffer from illusions forged via psychological trauma (which is well beyond the scope of this book), the majority of our ideas and ideals form from the mix of what we have inherited, experienced, and studied.

As many have said, *you don't know what you don't know.*

Further, *you won't know until you grow.*

Our grasp of reality is ever evolving. For example, if an infant could talk, she might say that "Mom is milk," and perhaps later that "Mom is hands and eyes." As a toddler, she could probably describe Mom head-to-toe as a distinct being. Yet she would still spend her life discovering—through hypothesis and correction or confirmation—Mom's personhood. Even after Mom dies, the child would still be pondering the complex depths of Mom and considering, with her own final breaths, much of Mom as a lovely mystery.

Strictly speaking, the infant's thought that "Mom is milk" is an illusion—an inaccurate idea. Yet, in all its inaccuracy, "Mom is milk" reflects the infant's healthy development. From birth to death, life is a continual shedding of illusions. Even spiritually, we awaken to God as children do to a parent. And regardless of how much time we are given on this earth, all that God really is will surely surprise us on the other side.

The apostle Paul acknowledged this reality in his first letter to the Corinthians: "Now we see but a poor reflection as in a mirror; then we shall see face to face. Now I know in part; then I shall know fully, even as I am fully known" (13:12).

Now we *know in part*. (Thank you, Paul.)

The rest is somewhat of a guess.

Personally, though, losing an illusion from a guess is far less painful than losing an illusion from what I thought I knew.

The problem is that we have a tendency to add on to truth by filling in the blank after what we "know in part." What we *assume* from what we know—rather than what we actually know—sets us up for the loss of a lot of illusions, especially when we confer upon our added-on assumption the spiritual weight of truth.

Like when we read, "God is love" (1 John 4:16) and then, consciously or unconsciously, add, *Which means that . . .*

He will protect me/my family from harm.

What is sincerely done in His name will be fruitful.

All who love Him should be able to love each other.

But then, a loved one has a terrible car accident, or we lose money on a risk we took in faith, or someone who once sincerely said "I do" is now angrily saying "I don't."

The Fall affects us all.

Yet we continue to expect Garden of Eden faith in a Garden of Gethsemane age. And without a framework for processing disillusionment, we treat our add-on assumptions as proof of what we know. So, for instance, if

God protects those we love from harm, then He is love. But if loved ones are harmed, then He is not love. Such reasoning gives more power to the add-on than to the truth. We wind up keeping the illusion (*I know how a loving God should behave*) and dissing the reality (*God is love*).

Valuing the process of disillusionment, however, does the reverse: it exposes our illusion as too small, too earthbound, and too simplistic to contain a supernatural and infinitely complex God.

If we think of God as the ultimate reality, then faith in God is a continual journey toward what is real. Along the way, life gifts us with opportunities to lose illusions and gain reality—neither as failure, nor as something demonic or punitive, but as healthy growing pains of spiritual maturation.

Which is perhaps why Paul encouraged the early church with, "Only let us live up to what we have attained" (Philippians 3:16). What a relief! We do not have to hold earlier versions of ourselves accountable for what our current version barely now knows! Returning to our previous example, we do not criticize the infant for not understanding that Mom is much, much more than milk.

So, if having illusions is natural and if disillusionment is actually an invitation to grow, why are we so tempted to bail in the process?

In *A Grief Observed*, C. S. Lewis offered the following insight:

> My idea of God is not a divine idea. It has to be shattered time after time. He shatters it Himself. He is the great iconoclast. Could we not almost say that this shattering is one of the marks of His presence? The Incarnation is the supreme example; it leaves all previous ideas of the Messiah in ruins. And most are "offended" by the iconoclasm; and blessed are those who are not.[2]

"Could we not almost say that this shattering is one of the marks of His presence?"

Indeed.

Reality is a merciful illusion-breaker, but the process can be deeply unsettling.[3] Why? Gerald G. May explains that, "since the night involves relinquishing attachments, it takes us beneath our denial into territory we are in the habit of avoiding."[4]

Resisting the night, we try to push it back with the feeble light of human understanding. Reason desperately attempts to hold faith in place, which is difficult to do when faith is growing. As Kierkegaard said in *Sickness unto Death*, faith "is precisely to lose one's understanding in order to win God."[5]

In other words, our greatest thoughts are still too small.

When in pain, we have to decide what we love more and what our faith is really in. Is our love and faith in God or in our understanding? (The former will always be too big for the latter.)

So, when that strong, loyal father dies suddenly of a heart attack, or a dear friend we have prayed for refuses to seek help, or we walk out of an appointment stunned by a diagnosis, a choice stands before us.

Will we trust God even when we do not understand God?

Are we willing to go without answers in order to go deeper into love?

Or will we label disillusionment a no-man's-land and bail?

John H. Coe describes how, when faith does not make sense, God is "purging [the believer] and inviting them into deeper fellowship with him."[6] This process summons us to surrender self.[7] We resist, in part, because we are rather attached to self and its illusions. So, in His mercy and through each night, God invites us further into reality.

He is bigger.

He is better.

He created us to be with Him.

And His companionship is enough, even in the night.

Chapter 8

. . .

THE UPWARD PULL
OF LOVE

It was Dad's companionship—not the roof over my head or the deck beneath my feet—that reframed night-storms as opportunities to strengthen and celebrate relationship. I found the courage to face the darkness because Dad was by my side. His love *for me* lit up the night *around me*. His calm presence made me fearless and even adventurous.

Without question, he could have made a different decision. His choice helped me grow through storms, instead of freezing in fear of them or anxiously searching for a way to avoid them altogether.

The choices we face in spiritual nights are rather similar. In the words of psychologist Peter Homans, in the night, a soul might:

> (1) move toward new knowledge of self, new ideals, and consequent new ideas, or (2) the paralysis can persist, leading to apathy, cynicism, and chronic discontent, or (3) one may disavow the experience entirely and instead attack, often fiercely and rebelliously, the events or persons producing the de-idealization.[1]

The third direction is an especially bitter version of bailing. The second direction, if maintained, can lead to theological despair. And the first direction—the discovery of new meaning—is where disillusionment becomes a true friend of intimacy with God and propels us upward into *love*.

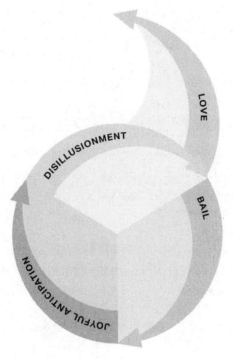

As night falls, we . . .
   "diss" illusions,
      gain reality,
         and begin to explore
         a greater depth of love.

Yes, of *love*.

Love is the treasure that awaits us in the night. And to be clear, I am not speaking of the feeling of love but the fact of love. Like faith and hope, love is not merely an emotion. Love is more like a muscle that becomes stronger the more you choose to use it. (And strengthening muscles does not always feel good.)

Love for God increases as it is exercised. In other words, the more you love, the more your love grows. And, like a healthy plant getting too big for its pot, a growing love will inevitably burst its current, comfortable container and expand to occupy previously unknown territory.

Giving God our love through the night grows us in ways that simply cannot be duplicated in the day. The night is among faith's most powerful purifiers and amplifiers of love *for* God. It is among the mightiest of mentors in living loved *by* God. Earlier generations wrote about this connection between night and love with greater frequency and passion. Consider, for example, this summary of the writings of a sixteenth-century Spanish friar, John of the Cross (1542–1591):

> In speaking of *la noche oscura*, the dark night of the soul, John is addressing something mysterious and unknown, but by no means sinister or evil. It is instead profoundly sacred and precious beyond all imagining. John says the dark night of the soul is "happy," "glad," "guiding," and full of "absolute grace." It is the secret way in which God not only liberates us from our attachments and idolatries, but also brings us to the realization of our true nature. The night is the means by which we find our heart's desire, our freedom for love.[2]

John of the Cross's perspective on darkness serves our focus well. He viewed the night as a sacred formational space. There is something about the dark that forges a love that is both rich (in grace) and resilient (through difficulties).

Such a love, as exemplified by Jesus, is not intimidated by pain. It grows in the midst of real, raw life. This is the treasure refined through disillusionment—a love that keeps increasing in strength and stability with each cycle as we lose more illusions, gain more reality, and choose again and again not to bail.

And love is what we really need, is it not? Love is the upward pull our souls long for. When drowning, whether in water or pain or confusion, we need someone, somewhere to pull us up. Sometimes I picture the upward pull of God's love as a divine magnet, lifting me to my true home. When we are disillusioned and choose love, our minds are drawn heavenward, and our souls move Godward.

As Gerald G. May states, "This deepening of love is the real purpose of the dark night of the soul."[3] Or, in the words of Coe, "The soul must learn to love God just for Himself in such a manner that He, and not the need to be loved, is the center of all things."[4]

Love is refined—it is made purer and richer—through trust. On those front porches over the years, the storms could be scary. But my trust for Dad outweighed what I could see and hear. In a similar way, by limiting human knowledge and control, the disillusionment process invites us to trust in God more than we trust in ourselves. C. S. Lewis speaks cleverly of the "moral beauty" of such trust:

> To love involves trusting the beloved beyond the evidence, even against much evidence. No man is our friend who believes in our good intentions only when they are proved. No man is our friend who will not be very slow to accept evidence against them. Such confidence, between one man and another, is in fact almost universally praised as a moral beauty, not blamed as a logical error. And the suspicious man is blamed for a meanness of character, not admired for the excellence of his logic.[5]

To trust—"even against much evidence"—is the inherent call of disillusionment.

Chapter 9

. . .

A CHOICE
IN THE DARK

Answers do not carry us through the night; love does.

The loss of illusions guides believers, in the words of Coe, "into the painful reality that apart from God, they can do nothing. . . . They are now ready for real love."[1] Our love becomes more and more *real* every time we move upward through the cycle of disillusionment.

Always, God's love is first. It precedes our existence, not to mention our faith. Then, like a sail that catches the wind of God's love, our choice to keep loving begins to move us forward. We love not because we know the future, but because God's very existence is weightier evidence than anything our eyes could perceive.

What, then, is the believer's responsibility when in spiritual pain? How do we move with grace through the loss of illusions?

The ability to journey from *joyful anticipation* through *disillusionment* into *love* is found in something relational, not informational.[2] In the night, God's presence in the darkness frees us to trust more, even when we know less. As May counsels,

The darkness, the holy unknowing that characterizes this freedom, is the opposite of confusion and ignorance. Confusion
happens when mystery is an enemy and we feel we must solve it
to master our destinies. And ignorance is not knowing that we
do not know. In the liberation of the night, we are freed from
having to figure things out, and we find delight in knowing that
we do not know.[3]

Mercifully, we are not alone in this journey through the dissing of illusions and the gaining of reality. Neither is our confidence in any "horizontal"[4] efforts. God Himself—not human optimism,[5] intellect, or
accomplishment—is pulling our faith upward into Himself and His love.

Unfortunately, on earth it is always easier to go down than to go up. The
upward pull of love is resisted by the downward pull of a fallen world.
One of the many challenges of the disillusioned state is that, though the
loss of illusions is a given, our *acceptance* of reality is not. It is possible to
prefer illusion over reality, resist love, and reject its accompanying offer
of intimacy with God.

The force that keeps us moving upward from *disillusionment* into *love*—
instead of downward from disillusionment into bail—is our *commitment*
to God.

Definitions of commitment abound. However, for our purposes, commitment is the act of "binding oneself . . . to a particular course of action,"
of "devoting oneself to something or someone."[6] To *commit* is to *keep
following Jesus.*

Throughout the Gospels, Jesus' "Follow me" never included GPS coordi-
nates. Following has always been more about *who* we are *with* than *where*
we are *going*.[7] This is why our trust muscles get more of a workout in the
night (when we cannot self-guide) than in the day (when we think we
can).[8]

Tragically, sometimes *commit* is the choice not taken. Yes, the enemy of our souls makes bailing easy and attractive. But we also can lose heart in the error that faith should always feel good. Disillusionment mercifully exposes that error. But staying committed to God through disillusionment takes effort. If we deem that work too costly and choose to bail, Rabbi Blumenthal cautions that the loss of illusions can end in the abandonment of religious beliefs.[9] To guard against such apostasy, Blumenthal offers the following guidance for processing the painful gaining of reality:

> Dealing with despair requires re-centering. Dealing with despair requires activating our anger and expressing our rage. . . . Protest—social protest, but also and perhaps more importantly, theological protest—is the first step. "Fear God"—in protest. Tremble, but say and pray the protest. . . . In a word, persistence in covenant. . . . Persistence, not hope. . . . I am not sure I hope, but I persist in the face of despair.[10]

Re-center + persist forge a fitting synonym for *commit*. Commitment is a willful, powerful force. In the midst of spiritual pain, commitment centers us in God, strengthens us to persist through the night, and then carries us into the upward pull of God's love.

One of the most vivid images of the power of commitment for me has been the adoption process. After a birth mother has placed her treasure in your arms, there is a window (often several weeks) within which she can change her mind for almost any reason. Though the option is protective for the biological family, the uncertainty can create a very vulnerable space for the adoptive family.

During one especially vulnerable experience, my emotions were all over the map. In my head, I knew that everything could change in a phone call and I was struggling with self-protection. But in my heart, I felt I had been chosen to be this child's forever mama and wanted to scoop up my baby and run for the hills. It was a night for me, and the uncertainty was relentlessly tormenting.

"How do you want me to steward this space, Jesus?" I cried.

His direction was clarion: "Don't shrink back, Alicia. Especially in the dark, commit to love this child 150%. Regardless of what the future holds, this child and you will benefit from all your love."

And so, I re-centered and persisted in giving my all to this child. Commitment—not certainty—carried me upward into love.

I do find it interesting that, in the context of spiritual despair, Blumenthal calls for "persistence, not hope." Perhaps he is referring to our tendency, in the community of faith, to inadvertently misuse *hope* to suppress honest grief, like a parenthesis that tames and contains its expression. Such efforts often truncate the grief process with an encouragement to place hope not in God, but in a better tomorrow around the corner.

In the adoption process, God did not dull my vulnerability with a sunny promise that the child would remain in my arms. He grew me with a principle that both the child and my soul would benefit from my commitment to love regardless of what the future held. Loving this baby as the overflow of living loved by God would make a powerful and permanent deposit in this life that no outcome could void. God comforted me not with, "Hold on, it will turn out like you want it to," but "Keep loving because I do."[11]

Biblically, hope in the night is anchored not in an earthly outcome, but in a Person. This is the hope exemplified by the persecuted saints listed in the latter half of the Hebrews 11 hall of faith, who responded to the painful gaining of reality with the power of commitment and "were all commended for their faith, yet none of them received what had been promised."[12]

Biblical hope is not a spiritualized form of positive thinking. Our real hope is not to just hold on optimistically until some brighter tomorrow replaces our darker today. Of course, we pray *for* relief, healing, restoration, and deliverance. But we must be careful not to hope *in* relief, healing, restoration, or deliverance. Our hope, biblically, is in a good and gracious God who is with us in every moment. His presence and love will accompany you and me through this life and into the next!

Jesus, the Person in which our hope is anchored, is a "man of sorrows, and familiar with suffering" (Isaiah 53:3). Which means that we do not have to wait for pain to pass before we can live today in biblical hope. Sowing commitment in the soil of disillusionment might be the most powerful spiritual weapon you and I possess.

A conversation between demons in C. S. Lewis's classic *The Screwtape Letters* pointedly speaks to this power: "Do not be deceived, Wormwood. Our cause is never more in danger than when a human, no longer desiring, but still intending, to do our Enemy's will, looks round upon a universe from which every trace of Him seems to have vanished, and asks why he has been forsaken, and still obeys."[13]

So, ask why, my friend.

Pour out your questions at God's feet.

Weep and mourn.

And commit, again and again, to keep following Jesus through the night.

Chapter 10

. . .

A SPIRITUAL EXFOLIATE

I find it fascinating that God designed some flowers to only bloom at night. Moonlight, not sunlight, triggers plants like evening primrose, moonflower, and night phlox to share their beauty and aroma. In a similar way, some aspects of love for God can only be exercised and displayed in the darkness. As Coe says so well, the dark awakens us to "the presence of the indwelling Lover of the soul."[1] How? By removing layers of a substance that hinders intimacy with God: *spiritual self-protection*.

Psychiatrist Anthony Reading explains that in relationships, "individuals who have been hurt by lost hopes tend to protect themselves against future disappointment by lowering their sights and dimming their aspirations."[2] Or, as an old saying goes: once bitten, twice shy.

One summer day I was bicycling around the neighborhood when two little dogs came running up to me. My experience with dogs up to that point had always been positive, so I smiled and thought, *How fun!* Slowing down to avoid running into them, I was shocked when they each sank their teeth into my legs. A rabies shot and several stitches later, my wounds eventually healed, but my newfound fear remained. For years, I was on alert and prepared to defend myself whenever a dog approached me. In self-protection, I distanced myself not only from potential pain, but also from the unconditional love that most dogs offer gladly.

The same can happen in our relationship with God. He does not bite, but life sure can. Shocked that God did not protect us from the pain, we easily isolate ourselves from Him. In self-protection, we distance our hearts from faith, hope, and even love to avoid further disappointment.

Spiritual self-protection refers to the many ways in which we consciously and unconsciously distance or hide ourselves from God.

The practice is not new. Adam and Eve hid "among the trees" (Genesis 3:8). We tend to hide in the weeds of distractions, denials, and details— anything to avoid the quiet, open spaces in which our doubts are deafening. Instead of entering the pain *with* God, we avoid the pain *and* God. Each choice to hide adds another layer that insulates our hearts from knowing the fullness of God's love.

Though the night is normal, spiritual self-protection is not. It is as old as the Fall but not as old as humanity. For an undisclosed era, we knew nothing of its burdens. Adam and Eve were spiritually formed through unguarded intimacy with God and each other. In the Garden of Eden, there was nothing to protect their "selves" from. Self was simply and profoundly *known*.

Then, when they ate the only forbidden thing in the Garden, they experienced a sudden impartation of the knowledge of good and evil, and "the eyes of both of them were opened, and they realized they were naked; so they sewed fig leaves together and made coverings for themselves" (Genesis 3:7). Though a fig tree provided the raw materials, shame volunteered as the first tailor. As Coe teaches,

> The first human experience after sin and the Fall was . . . *shame*, an "eye opening" experience of their own corruption or badness in the presence of one another. . . . The true distortion in their

nature, however, is seen in their first response to their shame: rather than fleeing to God for a solution to their problem, *they took it upon themselves* to find an appropriate cover for their disturbing nakedness.[3]

Adam and Eve's coverings were not sudden criticisms of their Creator's handiwork. Rather, such coverings were evidence of shame's contamination of all the eye could see. Though thin and light physically, the coverings were thick and heavy interpersonally. Shame now weighed down Adam's and Eve's spiritual formation, separating them from one another and from their God. Philip Yancey explains, "An awkward separation had crept in to spoil the intimacy. And every quiver of disappointment in our own relationship with God is an aftershock from their initial act of rebellion."[4]

Prior to the Fall, the "sound of the LORD God as he was walking in the garden in the cool of the day" (Genesis 3:8) was a spiritual formation summons to live in step with the One who gave all breath. Following the Fall, the same sound triggered an urgent need for concealment. In the words of Coe, "Human response to the existence of God is to imitate the first human couple, who feared the presence of God and hid from him (Genesis 3:8-10). These are the saddest verses in the Bible, for they mimic our penchant to hide from our maker, who alone is capable of loving us and opening us to true happiness."[5]

Hiding, obviously, hinders spiritual formation.

Any perceived distance from an omnipresent God is an illusion. However, the spiritual barriers created by the effort of hiding are all too real. Perhaps this feels familiar. Have you ever been so spiritually disappointed that you distanced your heart from hope or dialed back your personalization of God's love?

It is easy to hide in the night.

With the knowledge of good and evil, we no longer feel safe with God, with one another, or even with ourselves. Certainly, our interpersonal landscape has been shaped by this default.[6] Barring an intervention of grace, self-protection is self-perpetuating.

And unexpectedly, deliverance comes in the form of disillusionment.[7]

How? As we lose illusions and gain reality, each choice to commit to the upward call of love is simultaneously a choice to not self-protect—to not run and hide or cover and conceal. In this way, disillusionment acts like a spiritual exfoliate sloughing off layers of self-protection and leaving us more raw, sensitive, and vulnerable to God's love.

Some time ago, a brilliant leader whom I had the privilege of mentoring asked a pointed question on a disillusioning day: "Alicia, you speak of spiritual pain as a friend. But Satan's goal is pain. How then can it be a friend?"

To which I responded, "Great question. I don't think that Satan's goal is creating pain. I think that Satan's goal is creating distance. Toward that end, he can use pain or pleasure equally."

In the Garden of Eden, the serpent's agenda was (and still is) to create distance between humanity and God. With that as his goal, Adam and Eve's coverings and concealments—their layers of self-protection—were trophies to Satan. Our choice to commit to God's love in the night removes those layers and decreases our distance from God.

Disrupting the enemy's agenda of creating distance is one of the sacred works of the night. There, in the darkness, our deepest self-protective defaults are exposed, examined, and abandoned through spiritual pain.

So, when facing the night, my friend, do not bail.

Bloom.

There are colors of your intimacy with God, fragrances of your love for God, that can only be cultivated and released in the dark.

PART TWO

• • •

Disillusionment
with God

Chapter 11

. . .

YELLOW JACKETS

Have you ever been disillusioned *with God*?

If you are still reading, my guess is *yes*.

However, I have met a handful of souls whose answer was *never*. Although *never* can be a function of nature (hardwired personality), it seems most often to be an overflow of nurture (inherited theological frameworks). As far as potential spiritual health, there is a significant difference between *never questioning God* and *never being allowed to question God*. If you are in the latter camp, consider this encouragement:

> Leonard Sweet teaches that in the Jewish culture, "It's an act of reverence to ask questions of the story. . . . Around the table, a Jewish child has 'That's a good question!' drummed into his or her soul, not, 'You don't ask that question.' . . . Questions are as sacred as answers."[1]

> We weaken—not strengthen—our faith when we silence sincere questions. Faith in Christ is not an airy substance that rests on unquestioning souls. Biblical faith is muscular, thickened more through trials than ease.[2]

To strengthen our faith *in* God, we need to be honest when we are disillusioned *with* God.

So, be honest: Have your sincere assumptions about who God is, what God should do, and when God should do it ever collided painfully with reality?

Like Jay and his beautiful wife of two years, who were deeply in love and grateful for God's call on their lives. Heading back to seminary after Christmas break, their car slid on black ice and collided with an oncoming vehicle. Jay's bride died that day, along with all the dreams they had shared of a long life together.

Or like Rachel, from a family of witchcraft, whose life was gloriously transformed by Jesus. She grew rapidly in a community of faith in which a Bible study leader became her best friend and a pastor became like a father to her, until she found out that the two were having an affair. Then a new question tormented and threatened her newfound faith: *How could God let this happen?*

This is disillusionment. This is when we lose illusions and gain reality about life in God. This is when we truly feel the weight of God's words recorded in Isaiah 55:8-9: "'For my thoughts are not your thoughts, neither are your ways my ways,' declares the LORD. 'As the heavens are higher than the earth, so are my ways higher than your ways and my thoughts than your thoughts.'"

Well, evidently.

Even though the darkness may seem to hide God, through disillusionment, our God portraits are actually becoming more accurate. In the night, we realize that, though personal, God is not pliable; though a friend, God is not a peer; though loving, God is not confined by our logic. Through spiritual pain, God is revealed as more complex, which surely is a more faithful perspective. As the balloon pops once again, we are faced with a decision: Will we keep following Him? Will we commit, and, in the words of Blumenthal, *re-center* and *persist*?[3]

We begin our journeys with heartfelt words like "Jesus loves me, this I know." But those warm feelings can wane when dreams die, health fails, vision vaporizes, and we struggle to make sense of it all. Within those nights, our simple, sincere, and passionate praise *about God's love* gives way to a seasoned, sturdy, and more mature faith *in God's love* as we choose to echo Jesus' words from Mark 14:36: "*Abba*, Father, . . . everything is possible for you. Take this cup from me. Yet not what I will, but what you will."

Committing to this path of love when disillusioned is a sign that our faith is growing up. John of the Cross described this progression well, penning the following from a prison:

> At a certain point in the spiritual journey God will draw a person from the beginning stage to a more advanced stage. At this stage the person will begin to engage in religious exercises and grow deeper in the spiritual life. Such souls will likely experience what is called "the dark night of the soul." The "dark night" is when those persons lose all the pleasure that they once experienced in their devotional life. This happens because God wants to purify them and move them on to greater heights. . . . He will remove the previous consolation from the soul in order to teach it virtue and prevent it from developing vice.[4]

Though love-full, the process of spiritual maturity is rarely pain-free.

Our eldest, Jonathan, was diagnosed with autism at the age of two. We were told at the time that he might never be able to speak, let alone hold a conversation. To make a long story short, it took a village, and the journey still has challenges, but he did eventually speak, hold conversations, pass a high school equivalency test, and graduate from college (on the dean's list).

Though he was the eldest in age, Jonathan's baby sister Keona quickly assumed a position as his protector. I remember vividly one day when she came up to my office after Jonathan had been bullied at school. She was dressed in his clothes and stood there with her hands on her hips and said, "Nobody messes with my brother!" She wanted me to drive her to his school so she could be a shield between him and pain.

With his artist's soul and a wonderfully unique lens on life, chores were initially more about experience than efficiency. Some of our favorite memories include watching Jonathan learn to mow the lawn. At first, he went in circles, making designs on our few acres. We would all watch and smile, and then my husband Barry would go out and "just touch things up" after Jonathan got bored.

In time, though, Jonathan realized that another goal of mowing—besides artistic expression—was consistent coverage. Precision then became the game as he would go back and forth and back and forth, all the while singing some song at the top of his lungs.

One day, instead of singing, we all heard screaming. We looked out the window to see the riding mower unmanned, heading off a small cliff into the creek with Jonathan running in the opposite direction. He had mowed over a hidden nest of yellow jackets and was crying out in pain as more than a dozen stung him.

Ushering him safely inside, we tended to his welts and watched for reactions. When all was calm again, his protective little sister came to me with a burning question: "Why did God let that happen?"

"You're asking a good question," I replied. "You're asking why God allows pain. Some of the wisest souls throughout history have asked the same thing. What do you think? Why do you think God allows pain?"

Keona sat thoughtfully for quite some time. Then, with a sigh, she said, "Well, without pain, I guess we'd all be brats."

My little girl was disillusioned with God. Her courage to ask questions and her honesty to admit and address spiritual pain empowered her to make an early connection between suffering and character.

(Ah, the wisdom of a child.)[5]

Chapter 12

. . .

WHAT GOD WANTS

The frankness Keona displayed during the yellow jacket incident is a cultivated core value in our family. Close friends refer to our home as the house of emotional honesty. Though we try not to live in anticipation of drama, when it is our reality, we work hard to stay present to the pain together.

One such opportunity presented itself in the middle of my doctoral studies when an annual screening revealed a highly suspicious mass. The forty-eight hours between biopsy and the radiologist's call were unlike any I had ever experienced. A realist by nature, I knew that no one was guaranteed another breath. But in those two days of waiting, I felt my finiteness to a new degree. Looking into the eyes of my children, I ached thinking of what this might mean for them.

In the wait, true to our family value of emotional honesty, I asked my children how they were feeling. My eldest confessed that he had no feelings because we had no certain information yet. My youngest would not let me out of his sight. And my middle put her arms around me and said, "Well, if the biopsy comes back negative, God will be with us. If the biopsy comes back positive, God will be with us. So either way, we will be okay."

And there it is: ancient, biblical hope and commitment. With a framework for processing spiritual pain in place, I pray that such commitment-rich hope is rising within you and beginning to guide you through disillusioning times. Even when you cannot make sense of it, your spiritual pain is not senseless. God wastes nothing. Your disillusionment has been well-traveled by countless believers who have gone before you. And your commitment to the upward pull of love in the night is more powerful than you can imagine.

In walking with many souls over the years, general consensus exists as to what we seek when disillusioned:

Explanations: *How on earth did I get here?*

Deliverance: *How do I get out of here?*

Resolution: *How do I never come back here again?*

In the night, we search for understanding, freedom, and lasting change. However, motivations matter. They influence how and where we end.

When in spiritual pain, we are naturally motivated by what *we* want. But wisdom invites us to begin with a different question: What does *God* want? What is God looking for in the midst of our disillusionment? From His perspective, what would "success" look like as we navigate our nights?

Asking this question was a turning point for me. Well, more accurately, God asking me this question was a turning point for me. A long time ago, in a deeply disillusioning season, God and I had a conversation that went something like this:

Alicia: I can't figure it out, Lord. My brain and heart physically hurt from trying.

Jesus: *Alicia, what would be the height of success for you in this pain?*

Alicia: Resolution. A solution that returns the peace.

Jesus: *Yes, resolution is the treasure you seek. But it's not Mine.*

Alicia: You've got to be kidding. What could be more precious to You than peace?

Jesus: *Commitment to the way of love. What I'm looking for in you is commitment to Me.*

What?!

I thought God and I were working toward the same goal: ending the pain. Instead, "success," from His viewpoint, had less to do with my ability to change the scenery and more to do with my continued commitment to His company.

Oswald Chambers, in a teaching on the book of Job written for soldiers on the front lines, said that Job "never knew the preface to his story."[1] There was more going on than Job, at his best, could have ever figured out. The fullness of "why" was simply beyond him. And the same is true for us.

Yes, some troubles arise from the obvious, like when I was running up the stairs to save my daughter from an apocalyptic wasp, slipped, and broke my foot—no great mystery there. But when it comes to relational pain (with God, with our faith, and with others of faith), the preface to our disillusionment is rarely known in full. There are forces in play that are beyond our view. There are complexities at work that are beyond our comprehension. Chambers adds, "Reason is our guide among the facts of life, but it does not give us the explanation of them. Sin, suffering, and the book of God all bring a person to the realization that there is something wrong at the basis of life, and it cannot be put right by his reason."[2]

In the night, my treasure was *fixing things* through *figuring out things*. God's treasure was my *follow*.

This revelation is what inspired a statement I offered earlier: The force that leads us upward from *disillusionment* to *love* is *commitment*.

Through commitment, as we choose again and again to follow Jesus through the night, we *will* eventually find our way through the pain. Spiritual pain is not eternal. It is a temporary mentor—an unexpected friend of those who live a life of faith in a fallen world. Though the tools in the coming pages will help us navigate that night, we must remember that our commitment to keep moving upward toward love is more of a treasure to God than all our most brilliant solutions could ever be.

My longest night to date began with the words "I'm sorry." A little over forty-eight hours after the biopsy, the phone finally rang. I answered quickly, surprised by my sudden, rising hope for a good report. But instead of "all clear," the radiologist said, "This is not the news you were hoping for. . . ." My husband held me tight, and we called in the kids to talk and pray.

Some have asked if the cancer journey began my interest in disillusionment. No. My interest in (and study of) spiritual pain preceded that chapter by twenty years. The initial diagnosis was shocking but not disillusioning.

The fifth-year recurrence, however, was both.

It felt like a gut-punch. Cancer shifted in my mind from an unfortunate event to, well, a stalker. Jesus and I spent many years in that night together.

That sense of being stalked has, thankfully, faded a bit. The journey has, without question, shaped our family. Of course, I welcome your prayers. But I share all this to let you know that the tools I am offering have been collected by walking through, not around, many nights in my own faith (of which cancer has not remotely been the darkest).

Commitment to the upward pull of God's love is life—not mere poetry—to me.

Chapter 13

. . .

SOMETHING OLD

This ancient journey through the night is so important to God that He inspired writers to include in His Word story upon story of the painful gaining of reality. The most obvious books in the Bible to study pre-Christ examples of disillusionment with God would be Ecclesiastes and Job, both of which are among my favorites.[1] Instead, we will consider night-faith from the writings of a son of Korah found in Psalm 42.

I initially came across this psalm as a new follower of Jesus through a song inspired by its first verse. Soon after Jesus interrupted my atheistic existence, I attended a Bible college conference with one of the brave souls who had shared her faith in Jesus with me. During some session in the chapel, I heard a song that had been written right there on campus but would soon be sung around the world for decades to come.

Marty Nystrom, a schoolteacher by trade, found himself "broke and heartbroken" while visiting a friend in Texas. He entered into a fast and, on the nineteenth day of drinking only water, found an open Bible on an available piano and "God gave [him] a melody for Psalm 42:1. [He] just began to sing right off the page . . . literally."[2]

Marty shared the song with one friend, who shared it with the entire student body. The rest is history. Every time I heard "As the Deer Pants for the Water," it felt like my heart was lifted heavenward. The song brought (and can still bring) me to tears.[3]

The Scripture that inspired the song reads, "As the deer pants for streams of water, so my soul pants for you, O God" (Psalm 42:1). At the time, to me the verse meant that I loved God and wanted to love Him more; that He loved me and I longed to lean into His love more intensely; that I felt full but wanted to live a life that was overflowing. The sentence captured my heart's cry of, *Oh God, Your presence has satisfied my soul! But I desire to know You even more!*

Though not my main point, it is encouraging that God hears our hearts louder than our words. That is, He did not ask me to pause until I studied verses 2-13 before singing verse 1 with all my heart. Which is good news because it would be a couple of decades before I took a closer look at the rest of Psalm 42 and realized that "panting" is not pretty.

Panting is, in reality, rather stressful. It is an external manifestation of internal lack. Panting is caused when something is so essential that its absence leaves us in desperate need. Panting is about scarcity, not plenty; about mourning drought, not celebrating outpouring; about malady, not miracles.

In fact, the bulk of Psalm 42 is quite unsettling. Referencing himself (or perhaps the king), the author described his life as follows:

He was spiritually parched.

His satisfaction was delayed.

His thirst was unquenched.

Everywhere he looked it felt as though God were absent.

Tears were his food.

He was pouring out his soul.

He was experiencing a gap in the felt protection of God.

He felt forgotten by God.

He was mourning.

He was oppressed by the enemy.

He was being taunted by foes who appeared to be religious.

His soul was disturbed and downcast.

Psalm 42 is not about being spiritually satisfied at all! Psalm 42 is about spiritual pain.

Like countless souls before and since, this author's longing for spiritual growth led him into a season of disillusionment. Few—if any—in our day seek this. But if we want to grow in loving God, living loved by God, and loving others toward God, this psalmist's path will, at some point or even at many points in life, probably become familiar.

Though overlap exists in the types of disillusionment addressed, three lines in particular speak specifically to disillusionment with God:

My soul thirsts for God, for the living God. When can I go and meet with God?
PSALM 42:2

Deep calls to deep in the roar of your waterfalls; all your waves and breakers have swept over me.
PSALM 42:7

I say to God my Rock, "Why have you forgotten me? Why must I go about mourning, oppressed by the enemy?"
PSALM 42:9

Verses 2 and 9 require little interpretation: the author is expressing frustration over God's distance, physically and emotionally. The meaning of verse 7, however, has been a source of discussion for centuries.

Some have interpreted the images of *deep calling to deep* and *waves and breakers* as entirely allegorical, referring to spiritual intimacy with God. Spurgeon suggested that the image was connected to Genesis 1 as a picture of "the great deep above" connecting to "the great deep below."[4] However, current scholarship suggests that the image was probably inspired by the Jordan River at flood stage[5] and used here as a visual of wave upon wave of affliction sweeping over the author: "God is sending upon him one trouble after another. He is overwhelmed with a flood of misfortunes."[6] This agrees with how the verse is translated in *The Message*:

> Chaos calls to chaos,
>   to the tune of whitewater rapids.
> Your breaking surf, your thundering breakers
>   crash and crush me.
> PSALM 42:7

Crashed and crushed.

Like many honest souls in the Old Testament, this psalmist understood what it was like to be disillusioned with God. And, as we soon shall see, such disillusionment did not end when the New Testament began.

Chapter 14

. . .

SOMETHING NEW,
PART ONE

Several years after studying conflict in Scripture from Genesis to Revelation, I focused on a study of spiritual pain within the Gospels and realized that the disciples experienced a lot of disillusionment with Jesus. Their assumptions about who He was, what He would do, and when He would do it frequently collided with reality. Jesus kept bursting even their biggest and boldest balloons of preconceptions about the Messiah.

The instances of dissing illusions about Jesus seem to fall into three broad categories. First, the disciples were regularly disillusioned with Jesus' *timing*. For example, in Luke 7, Jesus comes upon the funeral of, by all accounts, a complete stranger:

> As he approached the town gate, a dead person was being carried out—the only son of his mother, and she was a widow. And a large crowd from the town was with her. When the Lord saw her, his heart went out to her and he said, "Don't cry." Then he went up and touched the coffin, and those carrying it stood still. He said, "Young man, I say to you, get up!" The dead man sat up and began to talk, and Jesus gave him back to his mother.
> LUKE 7:12-15

How amazing, moving, and confusing when you place this account alongside John 11.

> Now a man named Lazarus was sick. He was from Bethany, the village of Mary and her sister Martha. This Mary, whose brother Lazarus now lay sick, was the same one who poured perfume on the Lord and wiped his feet with her hair. So the sisters sent word to Jesus, "Lord, the one you love is sick." . . . Yet when he heard that Lazarus was sick, he stayed where he was two more days.
>
> JOHN 11:1-4, 6

Jesus raised a stranger from the dead (without anyone asking Him) and then delayed visiting a dying friend (even though loved ones reached out to Him). He raised an unnamed man in Nain and let beloved Lazarus die in Bethany.

No wonder we hear disillusionment dripping from the voices of first Martha and then Mary when Jesus arrived after Lazarus had already been in the tomb for four days. In succession, the sisters said the same thing: "Lord, if you had been here, my brother would not have died" (John 11:21, 32).

In other words, *Where were you?!*

Yes, unbeknownst to the sisters, Jesus was about to raise Lazarus from the dead, but perhaps one of the reasons we are unskilled in processing our own disillusionment is that we do not linger in the early disciples' disillusionment. We skip to the miracles in the Scriptures and expect to skip to the miracles in our lives. The space in between, however, is where love via commitment grows.

Another clarion example of disillusionment with Jesus' timing is recorded in both Matthew 8:23-25 and Mark:

That day when evening came, [Jesus] said to his disciples, "Let us go over to the other side." Leaving the crowd behind, they took him along just as he was, in the boat. There were also other boats with him. A furious squall came up, and the waves broke over the boat, so that it was nearly swamped. Jesus was in the stern, sleeping on a cushion. The disciples woke him and said to him, "Teacher, don't you care if we drown?"
MARK 4:35-38

Where were you? and *Don't you care if we drown?* are the cries of disillusioned souls.

Whereas the sisters' declaratives arose from sadness, the Twelves' interrogative arose, understandably, from fear: it is frightening when Jesus tells you to go somewhere and it looks like you are going to die on the way. To the sisters, Jesus was missing. To the disciples, Jesus was snoozing.

Both experiences are probably familiar to us. There are times when God seems utterly absent, and other times when God is obviously present but curiously unengaged, at least from our perspectives. Like when an innocent child suffers harm, a relationship is wounded by betrayal, or prayers for healing echo unanswered, and we wonder, *God, are You even here? If You are, why aren't You doing something about this?*

Though comprehending, let alone communicating, the complexity of God's timing is obviously beyond me, point of view seems a likely factor. Why? Because different points of reference can produce different perspectives about the same set of facts.

For example, my husband's family lived in North Dakota on the border of Canada. My family, in contrast, lived in Texas on the border of Mexico. Consider how these two different points of reference might interpret this set of facts: The month is April, and the temperature is 55 degrees Fahrenheit. These two states respond to the same temperature from rather different points of view. For North Dakota, this is a heat wave. For southern Texas, this is approaching an ice age.

In a similar way, we view time from a different point of view than God does. Our point of reference is today. Today we feel pain, today we know sorrow, today we need answers. Though God's point of reference includes today, it can never be contained by today. His point of reference is eternity.

God's grasp of time is immeasurably beyond us. His vantage point is higher than ours. We experience disillusionment because it feels like God is ignoring or overlooking us, but from an eternal perspective, He never does.

(Just ask Lazarus.)

Chapter 15

. . .

SOMETHING NEW, PART TWO

In addition to being disillusioned with Jesus' *timing*, the disciples were also disillusioned with Jesus' *words*. When reading through the Gospels, I picture the Twelve listening to Jesus' teachings, nodding their heads respectfully in public, and later turning to one another and saying, "Huh? Do you have any clue what He is talking about?" Here are a few examples with italics added for emphasis.

> The disciples came to him and asked, "*Why do you speak to the people in parables?*"
> MATTHEW 13:10

> When they came together in Galilee, he said to them, "The Son of Man is going to be betrayed into the hands of men. They will kill him, and on the third day he will be raised to life." And *the disciples were filled with grief.*
> MATTHEW 17:22-23

> When he was alone, the Twelve and the others around him *asked him about the parables.*
> MARK 4:10

On hearing it, many of his disciples said, "*This is a hard teaching. Who can accept it?*"
JOHN 6:60

Some of his disciples said to one another, "What does he mean by saying, 'In a little while you will see me no more, and then after a little while you will see me,' and 'Because I am going to the Father'?" They kept asking, "What does he mean by 'a little while'? *We don't understand what he is saying.*"
JOHN 16:17-18

One instance that always makes me smile is found in a confrontation between Jesus and some Pharisees and teachers of the law. After Jesus called these leaders *hypocrites* and rebuked them with searing words from the prophet Isaiah (see Matthew 15:8-9), His disciples came to Him and asked, "Do you know that the Pharisees were offended when they heard this?" (Matthew 15:12).

Can you imagine the guys huddling together before this intervention? I picture them strategizing a path to boost Jesus' waning image. Then, with confident concern, stating, "Lord, sometimes the way you word things is, well, rather harsh. We think more people would follow you if you talked less about sin. So, we've drawn up a PR plan that will help you present yourself with more woo and less woe. (You're welcome.)"

Perhaps we feel the same today when we read Jesus' words in John 14:6: "I am *the* way and *the* truth and *the* life" (emphasis added). In an effort to make our Jesus more attractive, we offer, "Lord, nowadays, people find the definite article *the* a wee bit too confining and intolerant. We'd like to suggest a slight adjustment from *the* to *a*. It will broaden your appeal."

Without question, Jesus' words—then and now—can offend. This is primarily because, in every age, Jesus is more concerned with truth than diplomacy. He is more devoted to reality than to illusions of peace.

Beyond being disillusioned with Jesus' *timing* and His *words*, the remaining examples of the disciples' disillusionment with God can be attributed to Jesus' *ways*. What He did, whom He called, how He spent His time, and where He went surely baffled even His closest followers.

> This is the God who welcomed children (see Matthew 19:13-15; Luke 18:15-17) and turned over tables in the Temple (see Matthew 21:12-13).

> This is the God who went out of His way to talk at length with a shunned woman by a well (see John 4:1-42) and yet refused to say even one word to a wealthy influencer (see Luke 23:8-9).

> This is the God who spoke tenderly to adulteresses while He skillfully humbled the religious righteous (see John 8:3-11).

> This is the God who protected those who rejected Him and corrected those who stood with Him (see Matthew 26:50-52).

> This is the God who exercised authority over the elements (see Mark 4:39-41) and yet let Himself be killed (see Matthew 26:53-54).

This is Jesus. And though His very breath sustains us, His timing, words, and ways can disillusion us. He does not operate within anticipated timetables. His speech and His silence do not correlate with anything predictable. What He does (and does not do) with His power is beyond our comprehension.

As I was studying, the early disciples' bewilderment, though surely uncomfortable for them then, was quite comforting to me now because it was *familiar*. Perhaps it is familiar to you, too.

Have challenging circumstances ever called into question Jesus' character? Have you ever been certain that the answer to a prayer was right around the corner and then rounded the bend to find yet another empty street? Have you ever wrestled with the why of unfulfilled longings or unexplained losses? Or have you ever just hung your head, like Jesus' confused disciples along the Emmaus road in Luke 24:21 and said, "But we had hoped that he was the one who was going to redeem [us]"?

Has it ever appeared to you, as it did to the first followers, that God just died?

What then? What can we do when the light of our faith in God flickers and seems to go out? In the next chapter, we will begin our consideration of nine tools to help us navigate disillusionment with God. For now, I offer a sweet story about flickering lights and trust in the night.

A long time ago on a warm summer day, we were visiting dear friends in their home. Our three children were thrilled to spend time with this fun family "in town." As far as address, their house was officially out of town on five spacious acres. But, from our kids' perspective, it was city living compared to how far out in the country we lived.

Barry and I chose our little house because of the old trees that surrounded it. The stunning sky at night and the glorious quiet of the countryside were unexpected bonuses. Over the years, we remodeled our home rather extensively, but the trees, the quiet, and the night sky have, thankfully, remained untouched.

All that to say that our three have grown up with darker nights than most of their peers.

While we were playing games at our friends' house after a great supper, the electricity suddenly flickered and then went completely out. Our friends' children were understandably startled and asked their parents if everything was okay. That is when I heard the clear voice of our youngest offering comfort in the dark. Five-year-old Louie said, "It's okay. The sun is still on."

True. Always, true.

When disillusioned, we too can be startled by the unexpected loss of light. But to paraphrase my now-not-so-little Louie, it is okay. The Light of the World still *is*, even when we cannot see, hear, or feel Him.

Chapter 16

. . .

GROWING PAINS

Our futures will be forged more by what we do with pain than by what we do with joy. This is one of the reasons why it is essential for us not to mistake disillusionment for failure. Such a misconception can incite us to bail right on the threshold of a growth spurt.

Growth, for all its positives, is still a form of pressure. By definition, growth requires change. Spiritually, that continuous growth is what keeps our faith, from its inception to its fulfillment, limber and flexible enough to follow Jesus wherever He leads.

And sometimes such growth leaves scars.

One day, one of my boys was changing his shirt, and I noticed a series of horizontal lines across his back. I stared at the uneven rows as my mind raced, trying to recall any accident that could account for the marks. There was no redness or sign of infection. It was baffling. How could something so new look so old? Picking up the phone to make an appointment, I was grateful for the regular checkup history we had with our physician. The next day in the clinic, the doctor examined my son's back and said, "Ah, these are stretch marks. A type of scarring that results from rapid development. He must have had quite a growth spurt since the last time I saw him."

Evidently, growth requires stretching.

(And stretching can leave a mark.)

Likewise, in disillusionment, our faith is stretched as it commits to the upward pull of love.

So how do we cooperate with such growth? How do we resist interpreting the marks as mistakes? What principles can guide us, and what choices can we make to keep following God through the night when He is the One with whom we are disillusioned?

A step-by-step, surefire plan for instantly dissolving disillusionment is way beyond me. It is beyond my head (I do not hold all the answers) as well as beyond my heart (for the health of your soul, I could never encourage you to sacrifice love for peace). What I can offer, however, are tools and truths that have helped many disillusioned souls (myself included) navigate the night with hope and grace.[1]

Many are understandably slow to acknowledge disillusionment with God. Often it can take years of processing disillusionment with self and others before a soul gives itself permission to direct disillusionment Godward. One friend explained, "I was actually proud to have never questioned God. I saw it as a sign that my faith was especially strong."

I still remember the moment she realized that, to keep growing, she had to start questioning. She had processed disillusionment with herself and with others but never with God. Even forming the sentence was painful for her. But when she finally blurted out, "I don't understand why an all-powerful, all-loving God would allow this," it was as though her honesty broke down an invisible dam of self-protection that had been blocking her growth. In the coming months I watched in awe as she found herself swept into a depth of God's love that had previously evaded her. My friend's discovery illustrates our first encouragement.

WHEN DISILLUSIONED WITH GOD, GOD IS NOT DISILLUSIONED WITH YOU.

God is the only one who has never had any illusions to lose.

As a beautiful song, "Jireh," says so well, "Wasn't holding You up so there's nothing I can do to let You down."[2] God has always seen you clearly and loved you fully. There is nothing you can say, nothing you can think, nowhere you can go emotionally or intellectually that can surprise or alarm Him.

God delights in your honest questions and even in your honest accusations. Because honesty with God—not just *about* God, but *with* God—is the antithesis of hiding *from* God.

Through spiritual honesty, we come out from Adam and Eve's trees, stand unprotected before our Maker, and in vulnerability, turn our tearstained faces toward Love.

So, for God's sake, just tell the truth.

Sometimes we spin our stories to relieve our theological angst. But making excuses for God cannot create intimacy with God. Chambers wrote insightfully in his study of Job about this tension: "Job's melancholy is the result of an intense facing of the things that have happened to him, and of his refusal to allow his religious beliefs to blind him to what he sees. Job refuses to tell a lie either for the honor of God or for his own comfort."[3]

Amen.

Hiding our disillusionment with God from God (and ourselves) is a colossal waste of energy. Further, sincere questions are not half as lethal to our faith as denied doubt.

Annually, I take an extended prayer retreat in Arizona. For hours each day, I walk with Jesus through a desert garden, pausing to journal and pray at the many stations of the cross. Canaan in the Desert is open sunup to sundown, and over the years, I have watched countless souls find refuge within its gates. Without question, the spot most often occupied is a bench that faces a close-to-life-size relief sculpture of Jesus draped in agony over a large rock at Gethsemane. A plaque nearby contains a quote from Basilea Schlink: "My Father, I do not understand you, but I trust you."

This is the essence of spiritual honesty.

An honesty that Jesus modeled for us all.

An honesty that could never cause God to be disillusioned with us.

Chapter 17

. . .

COOKIES
AND CANDOR

"What's the daughter thinking?" my dad would ask as we dipped yet another cookie in yet another glass of milk. His eyes would smile as I poured out my wonderings and worrying, my opinions and objections, my ideas and ideals. Early on, that sharing would include whatever dream I happened to have the night before and whatever stories a two-year-old could concoct. In my teens, our talks expanded to cover the pain of peer rejection and the headlines highlighted on *The Tonight Show*. As I grew into adulthood, Dad's standard discussion prompt opened the door for me to share about my joys and aches as a mom and my concerns and critics as a professional.

When Dad passed, he left me a rich inheritance, not of financial wealth but of emotional health. He gave me permission to ask questions, to express doubts, and to be brutally candid, *all in the name of love*. Though not a man of faith, by delighting in my honesty, Dad modeled a key truth about faith that has been a comfort to me through many nights.

WHEN DISILLUSIONED WITH GOD,
HONESTY PLACES YOU IN GOOD COMPANY.

One of my greatest prayers for you is that you will no longer feel alone in your nights. Many (myself included) are journeying with you. Our shared honesty about spiritual pain draws us closer together. (It is just that in the dark, it is sometimes hard to see one another.)

You are not isolated in experiencing disillusionment with God. Think of Job and his loss, Elijah and his depression, David and his discouragement, John the Baptist and his prison, the disciples and the Crucifixion, Paul and his thorn. Your disillusionment positions you squarely in their rather magnificent company.

In the Scriptures, world-changers were not shy about their disillusionment with God.

> Moses, who knew God face-to-face (see Exodus 33:11), cried, "Relent, O LORD! How long will it be? Have compassion on your servants!" (Psalm 90:13).

> Abraham boldly questioned God with the words, "Will you sweep away the righteous with the wicked?" (Genesis 18:23).

> David lamented, "How long must I wrestle with my thoughts and every day have sorrow in my heart?" (Psalm 13:2).

> Jeremiah pushed the envelope even further when he said, "You are always righteous, O LORD, when I bring a case before you. Yet I would speak with you about your justice: Why does the way of the wicked prosper? Why do all the faithless live at ease?" (Jeremiah 12:1).

Leaders, patriarchs, kings, and prophets all expressed disillusionment with God. And personally, beyond the Scriptures, just about every book I have ever wanted to read twice was written by someone familiar with the night. Our nights add depth to our days.

When we consider the disillusioned legends who have gone before us, it is clear that experiencing disillusionment with God is not our real problem. Our challenge arises from what we do *in* and *with* our disillusionment.

This second encouragement has a double meaning. Yes, spiritual pain places us in the company of the greats of faith. But spiritual pain also can enrich our experience of God's company. Paul called it fellowship,[1] which is a fruit of *follow-ship* with God through the night.

Relationship, not information, is the real gain of honesty. Company, more than data, is what our souls truly seek. Dad gave me the freedom to ask questions. But the point of asking questions was never finding answers; it was growing our relationship. I cannot remember even one answer to any of the countless questions Dad and I processed over the years. That was not the purpose. What I do remember is the safety of asking. I remember the comfort of closeness that honesty made possible. My questions were a means of deepening my connection with Dad.

The same is true spiritually.

Your honesty—even when it prompts you to question God's goodness—positions you in the amazing company of your heavenly Father. Because reality is a friend of intimacy with God.

Where we run into problems in disillusionment is when we process our pain away from God's company—when we isolate ourselves from His love through self-protection. Sometimes, when our beliefs are shaken by our realities, we withdraw from God instead of drawing nearer to God, hoping that the distance will somehow numb the pain. In actuality, the exact opposite occurs. As Oswald Chambers explained, "real suffering comes when a man's statement of his belief in God is divorced from his personal relationship to God."[2]

What is needed when we are in pain is to press in, not to pull back.

This is illustrated in the story of Mary and Martha, who kept their disillusionment uninfected by bringing their pain into the presence of Jesus. Martha "went out to meet him," looked Jesus straight in the eyes, and expressed her pain *to His face*. Mary "got up quickly," went out to Jesus, "fell at his feet," and poured out her pain *in His presence*. And Jesus responded by weeping with them (John 11:20-35).

Your honesty in the midst of spiritual pain not only places you in the good company of the saints who have gone before you, it positions you right next to the heart of the God who still goes with you!

Barry and I have tried to pass on Dad's legacy of emotional honesty to our children. Their whole lives, they have heard countless invitations to share their ideas, concerns, frustrations, dreams, plans, and disappointments. Listening to them, it is easy to understand why my dad's eyes always seemed to be smiling. We are hopeful that our children are inheriting a confidence that honesty about disillusionment is a means to growing their relationship with us and especially with their God.

Our daughter, Keona, was born dancing. She started ballet at the age of three, and by age fourteen, she had realistic hopes of dancing professionally after high school. That is, until our car was rear-ended at a stoplight. The first scans hinted at an L5 fracture, but they gave us no idea of the pain to come. After years of therapy, Keona's back pain persisted, but that paled in comparison with the pain of disappointment. By altering her flexibility, the accident had crushed a life dream. Keona was left with an ache in both her back and her heart.

Processing one night, I offered my girl the following: "Babe, you are really great at living *happy* with Jesus. And now you have the opportunity to live *sad* with Jesus. And that's okay because in the end, what will have made life rich will not be the happy or the sad; it will be the *with Jesus*."

In the brightest parts of the day and the darkest nights of the soul, *with Jesus* is always the best company we can ever keep.

Chapter 18

. . .

WHAT DOTS
ARE NOT

Besides the fact that it mirrors Jesus' primary model for growing people, I value mentoring because I daily taste its fruit in my own life. Well-placed words in a ripe moment can be revolutionary. Jesus, of course, is the master of this art, but His understudies have been used repeatedly in my faith walk as catalysts for growth.

One such moment occurred toward the end of my undergraduate studies. Becoming a lawyer had been my dream career since childhood. The grand plan after law school was to join a practice, simultaneously get a degree in computer science, focus for a season on computer law, and eventually enter public office. That plan remained intact until the beginning of my last year of university when it suddenly occurred to me that, since Jesus had done such a stellar job in saving me, I should probably ask Him if He had any preferences for my life post-college.

The query led me to spend one lunch a week in a quiet chapel just off campus to fast and wait on God for direction. The process was simple. With my journal and Bible in hand, I would take a seat on one of the wooden pews, voice my question ("God, what would You like me to do with my life?"), sit in the silence for five to ten minutes, and then read or worship. Week after week, month after month, I was discovering how God would often lead me. As I waited, some of the options became less substantial in His presence and floated away like dust. Other options gained substance in His presence and settled into my soul like foundation stones.

It seemed that God's "next" for me was to graduate and serve for a season overseas. So I paused my law school application (not knowing I would never loop back to it), announced my travel plans to my Texan parents (who kept hoping that "overseas" was code for Florida), applied to a missions organization, and sent out a newsletter inviting others to join me in this "step of faith."

All seemed well, until a campus pastor awakened me to an unhealthy pattern in my life through one well-placed discussion.

"Alicia," he began, "I've been concerned about something for a while now, but I wanted to pray before I said anything. I don't think that you walk by faith."

I sat there blinking, suppressing my urge to shout, *What? That's both rude and ridiculous. Do you see what I'm doing? I'm walking away from law school to go God-knows-where and eat God-knows-what so I can share Jesus with God-knows-who.* After taking a minute to compose myself, I responded (with more than a smidge of sarcasm), "Well, what do you think I walk by, if not faith?"

"Your understanding," he replied.

This was too much. I excused myself and left the table.

Somehow, along the way, I had learned that when someone you respect says something you do not like, you need to gather up the words, place them in God's presence, ask the Holy Spirit to blow upon them, and take to heart anything that remains. So back to the chapel I walked. Onto the altar the words went. Up to the heavens I sent a prayer of "Blow, Holy Spirit, blow!" And, to my horror, all the words remained after the wind died down.

God gently confirmed my pastor's words: *He's right, child. Do you know when you have faith? After you've considered a problem from all angles and finally had an "Aha!" That's when you become a woman of great faith. Until then, you're a soul in a desperate search for understanding. Have more confidence in the God who understands you than in your ability to understand.*

What God was teaching me in that space has been a powerful principle for me to this day.

WHEN DISILLUSIONED WITH GOD, THE KEY IS NOT CONNECTING THE DOTS.

Analytical by nature, I like connecting dots. Connecting dots calms me. But I dare not mistake the calm for faith. Faith is relational. When disillusioned, this distinction is critical. We can connect all the dots we want when disillusioned, but odds are, they will not coalesce to spell out *EXIT*. Intellect alone is a poor guide through the night.

In a personal diary chronicling his time in Egypt from 1915 to 1917, Oswald Chambers recounted a conversation with a noble dot-connecter:

> The other evening Mr. Swan was addressing some Christian Effendis[1] and called me over to tell them what I considered the real danger of theological training. I promptly said, "swelled head," and explained my belief that the only way to maintain spiritual life along with intellectual life was by the submission

of the intellect to Jesus Christ, and that then intellect became a splendid handmaiden of the Lord; that intellect should be the feet and not the head of the student.[2]

Disillusionment affords us plenty of opportunities to submit our intellect to Christ. God gave us brains. Clearly, He delights in our use of them. But thinking is not the same as trusting. And trust—with or without understanding—is how we follow God through the night.

In human development, our lives begin via God's breath, not our busy brain functioning. Which means that our spirits are older than our minds. Disillusionment reminds us to let the older lead the younger. We simply cannot think our way out of disillusionment, but we can give our trust-muscles a good workout by choosing to have more confidence in *who God is* than in our ability to connect all the dots.

Chapter 19

· · ·

THIRSTY THOUGHTS

Whereas intellect is a limited guide, God's Word is an unlimited source of insight. During my years as an atheist, I (obviously) disagreed. Optimistic Christians kept "gifting" me tiny, greenish Bibles. Culturally, regifting was not an option, so I stored the gifts in a restroom cabinet. Every once in a while, after devouring the latest *National Geographic*, I would pull out one of the little books out of sheer boredom, open it up, and see *nothing*. Of course I saw letters, but their meaning escaped me. The Bible's words seemed even thinner than the paper they were printed upon. *What nonsense*, I would mutter while returning the book to its tomb.

But after Jesus awakened me to Himself, all I wanted was a Bible. My very soul thirsted for one. And when I opened it up, I was shocked to discover that the Bible was not just a book; it was a Voice. All I wanted to do was hear, read, and study *that* Voice.

Except when I felt disillusioned.

When struggling with spiritual pain, I read less, studied less, memorized less, and interacted less with the Scriptures. Though understandable, it was the antithesis of what was needful.

WHEN DISILLUSIONED WITH GOD,
SOAK IN THE SCRIPTURES.

This is especially important when the Word is the last place we want to linger. Sometimes, when we are disillusioned, the Word seems to bounce off our minds like a ball off a wall. We can feel like hypocrites just going through religious motions. And if the Bible were merely a book, that might be true.

However, the Bible is a Voice that sounds throughout the ages. It describes itself as "living" and the testimony of billions agrees: "For the word of God is living and active. Sharper than any double-edged sword, it penetrates even to dividing soul and spirit, joints and marrow; it judges the thoughts and attitudes of the heart" (Hebrews 4:12, NIV).

Many books encourage. Many books instruct. Many books entertain. But this Book actually renews. This Book—the Bible—reads you.

And that is exactly what we need when we are disillusioned. In drought, plants need water. In spiritual pain, our thirsty minds need to soak in the Word of God. Every word we read, every sentence we listen to, every verse we speak aloud exposes our spirits to living water.

Choosing to saturate our thoughts with the Scriptures when we are disillusioned is evidence that our faith is based on *what is true*, not *what is felt*. Because the Word is living, continuing to expose ourselves to it when we feel nothing (and believe even less) is not hypocrisy; it is faith.

In fact, it is a lifeline.

Just before Jesus' arrest, He went with His disciples to Gethsemane. Positioning most of them toward the entrance, He took three—Peter, James, and John—farther into the garden. There, "he began to be sorrowful and troubled. Then he said to them, 'My soul is overwhelmed with sorrow to the point of death. Stay here and keep watch with me.' Going a little farther, he fell with his face to the ground and prayed" (Matthew 26:37-39).

When Jesus returned to the three, He found them sleeping. Matthew explains that "their eyes were heavy" (Matthew 26:43). Luke adds that they were "exhausted from sorrow" (Luke 22:45).

In other words, the disciples were disillusioned. Jesus' timing, words, and ways made no sense to them at all. Their emotions had been on a roller coaster as Jesus raised people from the dead but marched steadfastly to His own demise. Wearied with worry and fatigued by fear, they did what I do when disillusioned: they slept.

Jesus woke them up only once and gave them wise counsel for disillusioning days: "Watch and pray so that you will not fall into temptation. The spirit is willing, but the body is weak" (Matthew 26:41).

In his Gospel, John would later describe Jesus as follows: "In the beginning was the Word, and the Word was with God, and the Word was God. He was with God in the beginning. . . . The Word became flesh and made his dwelling among us" (John 1:1-2,14).

There, in the Garden of Gethsemane, Peter, James, and John were asked to watch and pray with the Word that had become flesh. Praying with the Word-made-flesh would protect them from temptation. Which is valuable, because when we are disillusioned, we are often more vulnerable to deception.

Like you, I wish I could physically grab hold of Jesus' hand to lead me through the night. But He has not abandoned us. He has given us His good Voice, the Scriptures, as a guide.

So keep reading and studying the Bible. Keep praying and memorizing the Word. Not because you feel like it, but because within His Voice is the strength you truly need to navigate the night.

Chapter 20

. . .

BODY BUILDING

Soaking our souls in the Word brings rest and strength to our spirits. When disillusioned, we need to be equally committed to the pursuit of rest and strength for our bodies.

**WHEN DISILLUSIONED WITH GOD,
ATTEND TO YOUR HEALTH.**

This encouragement is really about stewardship. Sometimes our health can take a hit in the night not because of the darkness, but from the fallout of our coping mechanisms.

Many of us instinctively go faster when disillusioned with God. In a vain effort to distract ourselves, we fill our days and flood our schedules with new undertakings. In doing so, we neglect self-care disciplines and binge on self-numbing activities. In our attempt to outrun the pain, we wind up running down our bodies with too little sleep, too little exercise, and poor nutrition.

Such avoidance is an utterly ineffective anesthetic for spiritual pain. It is like offering mud to a stuck truck in search of traction. A lot of energy is expended, but no ground is gained. Since a difference exists between relaxing and escaping, and since almost any activity could be rest for one soul and avoidance for another, emotional honesty is essential as we try to steward the space of disillusionment with God.

Others of us neglect our health in the night, not by speeding up but by slowing way down. When disillusioned, we do less . . . of everything. We move around less, interact with others less, pay less attention to what we eat, and inadvertently deprive our bodies of the fuel—sunshine, activity, good food, nurturing friendships, deep rest—they need to stay strong.

This is my challenge. My default in spiritual pain is to sit in a chair all day and think myself into exhaustion. One might see me and think, *Oh good, she's taking time to just be.* But *stationary* is not a certain synonym for *rest*.

When disillusioned, I have to will myself to make healthy choices. For example, I rarely fast when disillusioned and instead eat fresh, whole foods and drink a lot of water. Though I could easily stare out a window all day, I make myself take walks or play the piano. I find a truth-filled audiobook and let it fill my thoughts with something "other" while taking a detox bath. Or I hold hot tea in fabulous mugs and savor the snuggles of my family. All the while, my weary self slowly ceases its striving, and rest—health-inducing rest—refreshes me at levels that neither busyness nor paralysis are capable of reaching.

In the night, many speed up, others slow down, and a few, like Elijah, do a bit of both: they run fast and then crash hard.

On the back side of an epic high point in his ministry, Elijah slid into one of the lowest points of his life (which is not an uncommon occurrence among leaders). The prophet was about as disillusioned as a soul can get. "Elijah was afraid and ran for his life. When he came to Beersheba in Judah, he left his servant there, while he himself went a day's journey into the desert. He came to a broom tree, sat down under it and prayed that he might die. 'I have had enough, LORD,' he said. 'Take my life; I am no better than my ancestors'" (1 Kings 19:3-4).

The rest of the story reads like the notes of an infinitely patient nurse. God did not tell his son to *snap out of it* or *get over it* or *stop feeling sorry for himself.* Instead, God cared for him and let him sleep (verse 5), eat (verses 5-6), sleep again (verse 6), eat again (verses 7-8), take a forty-day road trip (verse 8), and sleep yet again (verse 9). Then, and only then, was Elijah able to identify and express his real frustration (verse 10) and hear God's voice in a gentle whisper (verse 12).

This pattern is worthy of adoption. When disillusioned with God, protect good sleep, eat nutritious food, move your body and travel (if possible), and be as honest with Him as you can.

Steward the space well by attending to your health with intentionality.

Chapter 21

. . .

IN THE
MOURNING

In disillusionment we lose illusions and gain reality. Something less accurate dies, and something more accurate rises to take its place. But since loss is still loss, mourning is still appropriate. Moving through disillusionment toward love does not mean that we do not grieve, but rather, that we process our sorrow sincerely with our Savior.

WHEN DISILLUSIONED WITH GOD,
GIVE YOURSELF PERMISSION TO GRIEVE.

When studying disillusionment with God throughout the Gospels, I lingered a long time in the space between Jesus' burial and resurrection. These were surely the darkest nights of the early disciples' lives. They had front-row seats to what history had been waiting for. They witnessed miracles and ate manna from heaven. And yet their greatest thoughts about Jesus were still too small.

Perhaps it was the thud of nails pounding into flesh and wood that canceled any remaining expectations of a miracle. Their illusions about who Jesus was were lost before Jesus' body was laid in the grave.

We too are familiar with the death of dreams.[1] We know what it is like to think that our dreams are God's dreams. To pray, believe, make plans, and work hard—and then, suddenly, it is all over.

Stunned, we sit graveside by lifeless hopes. And as we sit, we begin to doubt. *Did I miss something? Should I have prayed more or done more? Maybe I never really heard God in the first place. If this was not God's will, I must be incapable of knowing it.*

Jesus' disciples understood how we feel. They too had a dream that was cruelly crucified before their own eyes. They were certain their dream was God's dream, but then their hoped-for Messiah was murdered. Not even a fool could hope after that. The sealed tomb confirmed the truth: Jesus was dead.

Today we speed-read through these disillusioning days in the disciples' lives because we know that the joy of the resurrection is only a few verses away. But if we slow down, there is much to learn. What did they do after their dream died on the cross? How did they cope? What steps did they take to mourn the death of the greatest dream they had ever known?

> All those who knew him, including the women who had followed him from Galilee, stood at a distance, watching these things. Now there was a man named Joseph, a member of the Council, a good and upright man, who had not consented to their decision and action. He came from the Judean town of Arimathea and he was waiting for the kingdom of God. Going to Pilate, he asked for Jesus' body. Then he took it down, wrapped it in linen cloth and placed it in a tomb cut in the rock, one in which no one had yet been laid.
>
> LUKE 23:49-53

Speechless, Jesus' followers kept watch until the very end. They held on to flickering hope until its flame was extinguished. Then they gave themselves permission to bury their dream. After all, burial is a symbol of respect.

When dreams shatter, we too need to give ourselves time to gently collect the broken pieces and wrap them respectfully in tears. This is not about prematurely abandoning hope. This is about accepting reality. Denying Jesus' death would not return Him to the disciples. It was healthy for them to permit a burial. Faith is not threatened by funerals.

Then, the "women who had come with Jesus from Galilee followed Joseph and saw the tomb and how his body was laid in it. Then they went home and prepared spices and perfumes. But they rested on the Sabbath in obedience to the commandment" (Luke 23:55-56). Jesus' followers gathered by His tomb; then they returned home to prepare spices and oils to preserve and honor Him in His death.

Like the disciples, we need time to process loss when we are disillusioned. Those who have buried a loved one may need time to hold that person's favorite books or linger in their favorite chair. The entrepreneur may need unhurried days (instead of one angry hour) to reminisce as she packs up an office after an unsuccessful business venture. In response to that rejection letter, the student may need to head for the mountains to refresh his faith. Or the one who suffered a miscarriage may need to give herself permission to mourn instead of rushing to put everything away.

Take the time, my friend. Prepare the spices. Preserve and honor the memories. To echo our last encouragement, rest. Rest is essential—a need, not a luxury—when processing loss.

After the disciples rested, we read that "two of them were going to a village called Emmaus, about seven miles from Jerusalem. They were talking with each other about everything that had happened" (Luke 24:13-14). When dreams die, wisdom invites us to enjoy good talks and take long walks with trusted friends—just like the followers of Jesus did.

The disciples did not isolate themselves after Jesus' burial. They intentionally maintained their relationships. When we are disillusioned, we too must resist isolation. Even in loss—especially in loss—we are stronger together than alone.

Then, while "they talked and discussed these things with each other, Jesus himself came up and walked along with them; but they were kept from recognizing him" (Luke 24:15-16). The disciples did not know it, but as they walked with each other, Jesus walked with them. They could not comprehend it, but their dream, though dead, had not utterly perished! Its kernel survived and multiplied, just as Jesus had said: "Unless a kernel of wheat falls to the ground and dies, it remains only a single seed. But if it dies, it produces many seeds" (John 12:24).

Most of us will not see the resurrection of our dreams within three days. In fact, some of our dreams are sown for future generations to reap. Giving generously in the knowledge that harvest will arrive after we leave is a special kind of privilege and grief. But even then, our obedience is never a waste; it is an investment in a future we cannot see.

When we dream with God, even in disillusionment our dreams are not lost; they are planted. What grows from that painful planting is God's business. But sowing in faith is ours, and our faithfulness in the midst of disillusionment is never sown in vain.

Chapter 22

...

PROOF MISUSE

Oh, how my analytical soul loved writing proofs in geometry. All those neat, airtight, if-then statements connecting hypotheses with conclusions tidied up the planet with logic! In math, if-thens add clarity. But in faith, if-thens can create confusion.

Trying to explain the supernatural with one concise equation is like trying to explain the universe with one paper-thin dollar bill. The tools are out of sync with the tasks; the units of measurement are no match for the complexity of such dimensions.

Though this makes sense intellectually—though we agree that reducing faith to a formula is absurd—equations still sneak their way into our belief systems. They form in the shadows of our assumptions and are exposed—not by day, but by night.

WHEN DISILLUSIONED WITH GOD,
LISTEN FOR IF-THEN EQUATIONS HIDING IN YOUR FAITH.

I say "listen" because we most often hear such equations in our self-talk:

But I thought that if I _____, then God would _____.

If the Bible says _____, then I should receive _____.

If I am _____, then others will be _____.

If-thens are dangerous because they masquerade as truth. And untruth, if not identified and evaluated, has the power to undo belief.

I first began thinking about the power of spiritual if-thens when told a sad but true story long ago. Several families had covenanted together to be an active and practical community of faith in their city. They cared for their neighbors. They cared for each other. They gathered together to love and serve God.

The community grew as each member used their strengths to help whoever was in need. One such soul had an extreme gift of hospitality. Her home and heart were always open. Her hospitality was changing lives. With joy, she created warm, safe spaces for family, friends, strangers, and foster children in need. One child in particular won her heart. She began the long, red-tape-laden road of adoption full of confidence that God had brought them together to be a forever family.

But the courts decided differently and returned the child to a devastating situation. The helplessness was crushing. There was nothing she could do, no recourse or appeal she could make. The child who had won her heart was now out of her reach.

She walked around in a daze, numbed by a nightmare. Understandably, she did less than before, which seemed a healthy response to grief. But as the weeks and months passed, she became more and more isolated. She withdrew her help from her community and her presence from her family. Disillusionment descended into despair. And she bailed, leaving her spouse, children, and faith behind. She left, and, as far as I know, she never returned.

As a mom through the miracle of adoption, this story cut me to the core. I grieved for a woman, a family, and a child whose names I would never know. Yes, love is always a risk. Yes, spiritual warfare is no illusion. But I also wondered whether an *if-then* had helped set a snare for this hospitable soul.

Such equations can be configured in a variety of formations. Perhaps this mom's if-then was formatted as a statement: *If I serve God with all my might, then He will give me "the desires of [my] heart"* (Psalm 37:4). Or maybe her if-then was shaped more like a question: *Surely God would not have brought this child here if it was not His plan to keep her here, right?*

Our if-thens can be quite similar.

> *If God really loves me, then He won't let my heart be broken again.*
>
> *If God allows a door to open, then walking through it will bring me joy.*
>
> *If my dream is from God, then it will survive every storm.*
>
> *If my faith is strong enough, then I'll never experience depression.*

If-thens can sleep quietly, undetected for a long, long time until their slumber is disturbed by disillusionment. Once exposed, they must quickly be evaluated. Unprocessed, these equations can be catastrophic. Why? Because in some ways, our if-thens are really tests. Like children establishing criteria with which to measure the validity of their parents' love, our if-thens test God and then grade Him by our definition of goodness.

They do so by drawing straight lines between God's eternal character and an earthly, tangible outcome. Such simplifications cannot remotely account for the in-between layers and layers of complexities like the presence of free will, the mystery of spiritual warfare, and the reality of life in a fallen world.

So when our if-thens snap in two, we have a choice to make: Will we conclude that our faith is broken and God has failed us? Or will we diss our if-then illusions and join Jesus in the Garden of Gethsemane?

There with Jesus, in the night, we can fall on our faces and ask for the mountains to be moved: "Father, if you are willing, take this cup from me" (Luke 22:42).

There with Jesus, in the dark, we can elevate God's character above our understanding and add, "If it is not possible for this cup to be taken away unless I drink it, may your will be done" (Matthew 26:42).

Rereading the book of Job, I wonder if Satan was searching for if-then equations in Job's soul. The story reminds me of a scene in the first *Jurassic Park* movie (1993) when the velociraptors kept attacking the enclosure, and the game warden explained, "They were testing the fences for weaknesses systematically." In the first two chapters of Job, it is as though the enemy is testing Job's fences, systematically searching for weaknesses. *Will Job deny God if I press him here, with his wealth? How about here, with his children? Or maybe here, with his health? Perhaps here, with his marriage? Or surely here, with his reputation?*

Yet even Satan's most ancient strategies lose power in the presence of souls who, through the depths of their disillusionment, keep whispering of their God, "Though he slay me, yet will I hope in him" (Job 13:15).

So in the midst of our nights, when life breaks our if-thens into pieces, let us join Job in his loss and Jesus in His Gethsemane. When our logic proves itself too weak to hold reality, may we too lift our voices in prayer and say,

I trust You, my God, more than I trust my understanding.

I want You, my Lord, more than I want to avoid pain.

I don't need sight to have faith.

I just need You.

So lead on, my Savior.

May my faith grow stronger within Your shadow.

Chapter 23

. . .

A LIFELINE

Life is not tidy.

Unspeakable pain coexists with genuine joy.

Golden opportunity dances beside systemic injustice.

Shameless waste lives within mocking distance of abject poverty.

In the waiting room of real life,

one celebrates a birth,

another mourns a death.

One hears the word *benign*,

another hears the word *malignant*.

Real life is really complex.

Occasionally, Jesus-followers describe the gospel—the good news about God—as simple. However, *simple* is not a synonym for *accessible*.

Is the gospel simple? Perhaps. But God has never been and will never be simplistic. God never dilutes discrepancy nor ignores complexity. He does not conveniently edit out the uncomfortable. God is the ultimate realist. He is no stranger to pain.

Emily Dickinson said, "When Jesus tells us about his Father, we distrust him. When he shows us his Home, we turn away, but when he confides to us that he is 'acquainted with Grief,' we listen, for that also is an Acquaintance of our own."[1]

More than once over the years, my children have asked if Jesus is still experiencing pain today. I tend to think that He is.

Long before Jesus was born, Isaiah described God's servant as "despised and rejected by men, a man of sorrows, and familiar with suffering" (Isaiah 53:3). Though no longer on the cross, it does not seem to me that Jesus' heartaches have ceased. I cannot even begin to fathom what it would be like to see and hear everything being experienced by everyone on this fallen earth of ours. Surely, Jesus cares for us from within such world-size pain.

WHEN DISILLUSIONED WITH GOD,
ACTIVATE COMPASSION FROM WITHIN THE ACHE.

In the midst of our spiritual pain, we can follow this example of Jesus and care for others from within our pain. Caring for others when we are hurting can, at times, seem an insurmountable goal. But when we are disillusioned, activating even a little bit of compassion can serve to guard our emotional and mental well-being.

The image of a waterwheel comes to mind. In some ways, a waterwheel is a protest against wasted potential. Placed in a river vertically or horizontally, the wheel harnesses the energy of a moving body of water to do something productive, like grind grain or power machinery. Unlike a dam, the wheel does not store up the water; it simply refuses to let the water go by without making a positive contribution. We too can refuse to let the disillusionment pass by without activating something within us to help others.

The *Oxford English Dictionary* defines *activate* as "to make (more) active; to move to activity; to initiate (a process). Also: to motivate."[2] Activation does not create something from nothing; it calls something that already exists into action.

Calling our compassion into action is crucial when we are disillusioned. Spiritual pain sensitizes us to every kind of pain. If we only attend to our own pain when disillusioned, it may overwhelm us. But if we lift up our heads and look around, we can harness the power of pain in our own lives to make a positive difference in others' lives.

That is exactly what a beautiful soul named Josette did for me.

Somehow, Josette read a book I wrote and sent it to her sister, Michelle. When Michelle read the book, she reached out to me and quickly became a dear and trusted friend. She and her husband were among those surrounding us in prayer during the fifth-year cancer recurrence that took our family completely by surprise.

A researcher by nature, once the initial shock and mental paralysis began to subside, I embarked on a deep dive into traditional and nontraditional treatment possibilities and nutritional approaches for recurrences and quickly became overwhelmed. I needed a mentor through the night. God provided abundantly as Michelle introduced me to Josette, the sister who had introduced Michelle to me!

Josette was a brilliant guide. In the three years since her own cancer diagnosis, she had processed more research than I thought imaginable. Phone call after phone call, Josette listened intently as I poured out my questions and confusion. She patiently and generously offered her expertise with a calming combination of objectivity and compassion. Josette shared everything, sold nothing, and trusted God to ultimately guide me.

What neither of us knew when we began our friendship was that she had mere months to live.

Though neither of us feared death, we both were fighting to live as long and as strong as we could for the sake of our children. Below are excerpts from our final texts just days before Josette went Home. Listen for the spiritual strength and emotional honesty sounding from within her physical pain:*

DECEMBER 14

Alicia: How are you? You're on my heart today. Praying for you!

Josette: There's a definite reason I am on your heart. I declined really fast and when we got to the hospital, we were told that my liver has much more cancer than they thought. They made it sound VERY hopeless. I went to bed that night feeling scared, unsure, etc. I'm physically still struggling but I am at peace and have my hope back. I can't tell you what it means to me that you are checking on me and praying. I'm so grateful. Prayer is what we need. It's been over 3.5 years and we are tired. We need people to hold our arms up at this point. I hope and pray that you are doing well!!!

Alicia: You are in my prayers. I'm so grateful for your encouragement and all that you've shared with me. Love and prayers and hope eternal!

DECEMBER 17

Alicia: Love you, my friend. I woke up early this morning and prayed for you.

---

*This text trail is shared with permission of Josette's sister, Michelle.

Josette: Alicia, you waking and praying for me was beyond timely. Was put back in the hospital this morning and am told we have to make the hard decisions now. God woke several significant people in my life this morning. As grueling as the hard talks were today, I literally felt carried. I became so overwhelmed by the thought of the God of the universe loving me enough to give His undivided attention to my needs, it brought me to tears. I don't know what else to say but thank you!!!!!!

Alicia: Oh yes—He treasures you! I had several thoughts while praying for you but I was overwhelmed by one in particular. Josette, your faithful, consistent choice to love God in all things (each valley, every mountaintop, and every step in between) has forged a spiritual inheritance FOR YOUR SON that will shape him and crown him and protect him. Your love—Josette's love for Jesus—is a powerful force for God and for good. The real fight on this earth isn't for health, it's for love. Whatever the doctors are saying, you won the real battle long ago. Well done, great and mighty lover of God!!! I continue to stand with you in prayer and hope!

DECEMBER 18
Josette: This speaks to my soul in a way I cannot really express. Thank you for continuing to pray and stand with us

There was no period at the end of Josette's last sentence to me. I found its absence comforting. We will pick up our conversation when we see each other again. The advice Josette gave to me, especially in her last weeks, has continued to guide me to this day. She was fighting for her life, stalked by an aggressive cancer, yet she reached into her ache and activated compassion for me and many others.

In our talks, Josette spoke of her longing to write a book about what she had learned so that her experience could help others. She did write one, but on human hearts instead of paper pages. Her words live on in souls like mine that she compassionately cared for until the very end.

Likewise, our compassion does not have to be packaged into something formal in order to be fruitful. Any effort, however plain or simple it may seem, can be immensely meaningful when offered in love.

So when in spiritual pain, text "Thinking of you!" to a friend or write an encouraging note to a former teacher. Give some "ice cream money"[3] to a struggling college student or tell a teen that their life makes the world a better place. Send a lonely soul some flowers or donate clothes to a shelter or food to a pantry.

In your nights, invest in acts of compassion.

They will strengthen others and be a lifeline of sanity for you.

Chapter 24

. . .

THE
UNGLAMOROUS
GIFT

Writing of her experience at a conference, Kathleen Norris recounted the following moving story:

> Near the end of a recent Monastic Institute . . . an anguished young Trappist spoke up: "We've spoken of the loss of faith in American society. But what of loss of faith within the monastery itself?" He indicated that he was living, as a monk, with profound doubts, and that while the monastery was where he felt he belonged, at times his life there was nearly unbearable. Fr. Lafont nodded; none of this, evidently, was a surprise to him. What he said in response struck me as both practical and thoroughly monastic: "Of course we are weak, unable to cope. But if we can maintain faith, hope, and charity, it will radiate somehow. And people who come to us may find in us what we can no longer see in ourselves."[1]

This last sentence strikes me as profound. In the midst of spiritual pain, if we keep moving Godward, if we commit to the upward pull of love, others near us may "find in us what we can no longer see in ourselves": faith, hope, and love. In other words,

WHEN DISILLUSIONED WITH GOD, PLOD ON.

My favorite genres of books are history and memoir. I especially love biographies and, early in my faith journey, invested untold hours reading the stories of missionaries. This is when the expression *plod on* took on new meaning for me.

I read the phrase in a self-description of William Carey (1761–1834). A British minister considered to be the founder of modern missions, Carey was intimately familiar with loss. Within his first year in India, his son died of illness and his wife, Dorothy, experienced a breakdown from which she never recovered. He would eventually bury two wives in his adopted land.

Carey did not witness a decision to follow Christ among those he served until his seventh year in the country. In addition to establishing Serampore College and organizing the Agricultural Society of India, Carey translated the New Testament into Bengali, published a New Testament in Sanskrit, wrote grammars in Bengali, Sanskrit, and Marathi, translated Indian literature into English, taught as a professor on the subjects of divinity, botany, and zoology, and helped establish India's first printing press![2]

Clearly, Carey spent his days surrounded by a lot of paper—paper that represented his life's blood, work, and tears. Then, in March of 1812, much of Carey's labor of love went up in flames when a room at the printing press—filled with twelve thousand reams of stored paper—caught on fire. Irreplaceable works, including grammars, presses, manuscripts, dictionaries, and ten translations of the Bible typeset for printing in fourteen languages, were turned to ash. As Carey would write to a friend, "The loss is heavy."[3]

That evening, Carey came to survey the incalculable damage. And then he picked up a pen and started again.

Imagine.

Later on, Carey said the following: "If, after my removal, anyone should think it worth his while to write my life, I will give you a criterion by which you may judge of its correctness. If he gives me credit for being a plodder, he will describe me justly. Anything beyond this will be too much. I can plod. I can persevere in any definite pursuit. To this I owe everything."[4]

At first glance (and even at second glance) a call to *plod* can sound less than inspiring. It means "to work steadily and laboriously, or in a stolid or monotonous fashion; to drudge or toil."[5]

Fantastic.

But if we were to peel back history and examine the origin stories of some of its greatest inventions, accomplishments, and contributions, we might have more appreciation for this unglamorous gift of plod. We would see Thomas Edison plodding through his oft-quoted "ten thousand ways that will not work" on his road to innovation, of whom a biographer said, "Edison's not a guy that looks back. Even for his biggest failures he didn't spend a lot of time wringing his hands."[6] We would see Nelson Mandela plodding through twenty-seven years in prison before becoming the first Black president of South Africa and later saying of himself, "I was not a messiah, but an ordinary man who had become a leader because of extraordinary circumstances."[7] But above all, we would see Jesus (who *was* the Messiah), plodding His way past misunderstanding and rejection to and through the cross: "As the time approached for him to be taken up to heaven, Jesus resolutely set out for Jerusalem" (Luke 9:51).

Spiritually, *plodding* is about moving forward, not by leaps and bounds over tall buildings, but by choices and tears through pain-filled nights.

Plodding is about leaning Godward even when we feel like we are standing still or falling backward.

Plodding (like *re-centering* + *persisting*) is a worthy synonym for *commitment*.

And *commitment* is the path that pulls us upward from disillusionment into love.

Chapter 25

• • •

ON THE
OTHER SIDE

Our focus in Part Two has been disillusionment with God—when we experience the painful gaining of reality about our Creator. My prayer is that these chapters have been both freeing and comforting. That they have somehow given you permission to be honest about spiritual pain in the confidence that your nights are a sign that your faith is growing, not retreating.

In the midst of your disillusionment with God, remember:

God is not disillusioned with you.

Honesty about the pain places you in good company.

The key is not in your ability to connect the dots.

Instead, soak in the Scriptures.

Attend to your health.

Give yourself permission to grieve.

Listen for if-then equations.

Activate your compassion.

And . . .

Plod on.

Plod on . . . *Toward what?*

Toward love—God's love for you and your love for Him.

Plod on . . . *Why?*

Because you and your faith are irreplaceable. Your commitment to follow Jesus, especially through the night, is a powerful weapon against the forces of evil on this earth.

Earlier, I shared the story of a couple whose car slid on black ice on their way back to seminary. Jay did not find out that his wife had died in the crash until a full day after the accident. Road conditions prevented family from coming to the hospital right away, so he heard of his wife's passing from a local pastor who said softly, "Son, she's with the Lord."

The young widower's hands shot up in the air, and from his gut he found himself saying, "Welcome her for me, Jesus! Tell her that I love her!" Jay wept with the pastor by his side, overcome by God's presence.

The coming days and years would be much darker. The loss was overwhelming. Often, Jay wondered why God had not taken him as well. Later he explained, "When you bury someone you love, it's like 90 percent of yourself is buried too." Advised to do the last thing he heard God say, the young man returned to seminary and to his classes, including one he had already enrolled in called "Grief, Death, and Dying."

In short, Jay plodded on.

Rachel—from the other story in chapter 11 about a young woman who came to Jesus from a background of witchcraft—did not. The shock over the affair between her Bible study leader and her pastor soon gave way to sadness and anger, all of which were healthy steps in the grief process. Grief did not lead her to bail; bitterness did. The betrayal was bad enough, but the injustice of how it was all handled was simply too much.

And so, she denied the existence of a God who could let such a tragedy occur. She denounced the faith that had miraculously freed her from demonic powers. She rejected the broken body of Christ that had imperfectly addressed the affair and its fallout.

When entering nights this deep, both these paths stand before us: one that defies gravity and moves upward toward love and another that surrenders to gravity and bails. Interestingly, both paths can, at first, sound identical as we hold the pain in our hands, look up to the heavens, and yell, "Well, Jesus, surely an all-powerful God could have prevented this. But You didn't."

What separates these two paths is whether we end this cry with a period or with a comma.

When ended with a period, we draw the pain more deeply into our souls, turn our backs toward the God who disappointed us, walk away, and bail.

But when honesty about our pain is followed by a comma, our first cry is followed by a second cry: "However, 'to whom shall we go' but to you?" (see John 6:68).

In other words, we take our pain and turn toward God.

We take our pain and press it into His heart.

We take our pain and plod on.

Instead of bailing, we commit to the upward pull of love.

What God does in such souls is extraordinary. There is a quality among those who choose this way of love that, though hard to quantify, is unmistakable. A scent of heaven mingling with the tears of earth; a richness of character that can neither be feigned nor fabricated.

Six years after Jay's wife died, I heard his story at a retreat in which we were placed in the same small group. The loss had scarred him, but his choice to keep loving God had shaped him. In fact, it shaped him into the man I fell in love with and eventually married.

Barry Jay Chole has been my love, best friend, champion, and chief encourager ever since. Our three children through the miracle of adoption have one of the best dads on the planet because Barry committed to the upward pull of love when disillusioned by the loss of his beautiful first wife.

My friend, never underestimate what or who is awaiting you on the other side of your disillusionment. More depends on your choice to keep loving God than you can imagine. The destiny of nations could rest on the choices you make today in the depth of the night.

What would have become of God's people if Joseph had refused to plod on through being misunderstood and falsely accused? What would our Bibles look like if the prophets had decided to stop speaking because it did not seem to make any tangible difference? What would have happened to the early church if Paul had given up writing, unable to press past disillusionment from the opposition that surrounded him?

Where would you and I be if the person who led us to Jesus had abandoned faith when they felt depressed? Or become bitter when they lost their job? Or withdrawn from God when their loved one died? Or bailed because they were betrayed?

To us is given the responsibility of building the bridge of faith toward the next generation.

One brief glance at the crucifixion assures us that construction must continue *especially* in the night.

No matter how dark it may seem in your life right now, your Savior is with you! He stands right beside you, holding you in the midst of your storm. This night will not last forever, but the faith you place in Him in this moment will echo into the future, making the way for generations to come!

PART THREE

Disillusionment with Self

Chapter 26

...

SPIRITUAL FRUSTRATION

When a child falls while learning to ride a bike.

When a successful high school student is stunned by their first college C.

When a sleep-deprived new parent is at their wit's end.

When a professional prepares well but presents poorly.

When an always-active soul has to come to terms with decreased strength.

Every season of life grants all who breathe the opportunity to lose illusions about themselves. Though it is a common human experience, our focus will be disillusionment with self *in the life of faith*. This is a distinctly spiritual application. This is when expectations of what we can and will do as followers of Jesus collide painfully with reality.

Walking with God throws open otherwise-impossible doors for soul-deep change. Truly, "if anyone is in Christ, he is a new creation; the old has gone, the new has come" (2 Corinthians 5:17). Being new is a given for those who believe. However, walking out that newness almost always initiates disillusionment about our humanity, in general, and our faith, in particular.

Disillusionment with self is when we wonder . . .

> *How could I have done that? I knew better.*
>
> *I used to feel God's presence. Now, I feel nothing at all.*
>
> *I thought this is what God told me to do. Evidently, I was wrong.*
>
> *Why won't this anxiety/fear/sadness go away? I can't seem to shake it.*
>
> *Aren't I supposed to be "more than a conqueror"? Why, then, am I still so defeated?*

The temptation to bail in this type of spiritual pain lies not in a loss of faith in God, but in a loss of confidence in our ability to follow God. Instead of "I thought that *God* would be different," disillusionment with self prompts us to whisper, "I thought that *I* would be different."

It is a form of spiritual frustration.

Frustration refers to "the feeling of being upset or annoyed, especially because of inability to change or achieve something."[1] In the context of disillusionment, frustration is an emotional response to spiritual impotence.

According to the *Oxford English Dictionary*, the verb *frustrate* made its first appearance in 1447,[2] while the noun *frustration* appeared some 128 years later in 1575.[3] The word comes to us from the Latin root *frustrari*, which means "to deceive or disappoint."[4]

Being disappointed as a linguistic root for frustration made sense to me, but *being deceived*? How is frustration related to deception? I found the connection intriguing, and after a bit more thinking, it too made sense.

Frustration is the feeling we have when *our expectations deceive us*—when there is a gap between our starting outlook and our current outcome.

A relatively benign example of this might be when a friend tells you to see a movie because it is "the best thing ever." If your high expectations are not upheld by the actual experience, in the letdown you may wonder why your friend oversold the show. Beyond feeling disappointed, you might feel a bit *misled*.

In daily living, frustration is not uncommon. We feel it when we have just enough time to get to an appointment, hop in the car, and remember that it is almost out of gas. Or when we spend an hour on hold waiting to talk with a human only to be told that we called the wrong department and be placed on hold again.

But spiritual frustration can be very confusing. It is one thing to feel misled by a friend's overly optimistic review, by our own forgetfulness to fill the tank, or by an "anti-helpful"[5] automated customer service system. It is another thing entirely to feel misled—or even deceived—by faith-inspired hopes. This is why *frustration* is an apt word to use when disillusioned with ourselves.

Have you ever felt let down by what you thought were reasonable, Bible-based expectations? Perhaps that all your weaknesses would be replaced by strengths? That impossible plans would miraculously come to pass? That the sea would somehow part? That you would wake up and be free from bitterness in your heart?

This is what happens when . . .

> Your godly character is more godly at work than at home.
>
> Your sincere desire to keep people happy is keeping you alarmingly exhausted.
>
> Memorizing the Word has not freed you from being held hostage by bad memories.

You thought you were making progress, until that one person said that one thing.

Paul's advice in Colossians 3:2 to "set your [mind] on things above" does not seem to be immunizing you to the toxicity of things below.

If not identified and processed, disillusionment with self can end in a brokenhearted bail "for God's sake" (e.g., *I don't want to shame God's name any longer with my failures*) or even a coldhearted discarding of faith (*It didn't work for me. I wonder if it really works for anyone*).

In the same way that God is not disillusioned with us when we are disillusioned with Him, He is not disillusioned with us when we are disillusioned with ourselves. Unlike us, He has never been under any illusions about our faith or our humanity. He knows full well how the Fall affects us all. And He stands ready to mentor us through the painful gaining of reality about ourselves. As David said in Psalm 103:14, "For he knows how we are formed, he remembers that we are dust."

Seeing ourselves as dust, however, can be painful. Committing to God in the midst of that pain will require us to value His presence more than our quantifiable progress.

Thankfully, many sincere and vulnerable souls have already shown us the way.

Chapter 27

. . .

SOMETHING OLD

From David's "Surely I was sinful at birth" (Psalm 51:5) to the disciples' "Surely not I, Lord?" (Matthew 26:22), examples of disillusionment with self are not difficult to find in the Scriptures. Returning to Psalm 42, one phrase in particular captures this sense of spiritual self-frustration especially well: "Why, my soul, are you downcast? Why so disturbed within me? Put your hope in God, for I will yet praise him, my Savior and my God" (Psalm 42:5, 11).

The author repeats this refrain verbatim at the end of the psalm. When considering this repetition, we often focus on the psalmist's healthy habit of speaking truth to his soul. Though that discipline is unquestionably powerful, what always catches my interest in this psalm is the son of Korah's frustration that his emotions were not reflecting his beliefs. If you will permit a paraphrase, perhaps he was saying, "I *know* what's true! Why isn't that changing how I *feel*?"

His angst is familiar to me, but that is a relatively recent development.

One of my first original teaching illustrations was a simple drawing of an even simpler train that had three cars labeled (in order) *feelings*, *truth*, and *will*. Teaching from Romans 12:2—"Do not conform to the pattern of this world, but be transformed by the renewing of your mind"—I used the image to portray how one of the world's patterns is to determine truth through the leadership of our emotions (i.e., *Do I feel it? Then it's true.*).

After layering multiple examples of how this pattern played out in our lives, I would rearrange the cars, placing *truth* in the lead, *will* next, and *feelings* last. Then I'd say something like this:

> Though unqualified to lead, please note that we don't leave feelings at the depot. I like feelings, especially when they reflect truth. When they don't, though uncomfortable, it is still livable. They're at the end of the train, and they're coming with me anyway. In fact, they are welcome to drag their fickle little feet behind truth all the way to heaven.[1]

The illustration has served my walk well. It has helped me acknowledge and honestly attend to my emotions, while recognizing that, though real, they may not be true.

Why the backstory? To relay that, for a long time, I have been aware that emotions do not politely line up behind truth as soon as it is uttered. The existence of a discrepancy between what I know and how I feel is both logical and anticipated. Nonetheless, that discrepancy still proved to be close to unbearable a few years ago.

I mentioned earlier that the fifth-year cancer recurrence felt like a punch to the gut. This was not because I had some "word from the Lord" that cancer was behind me. Actually, I had something much more convincing for my wiring: I had *peace*.

Going into that fifth-year scan, there was not an atom of fear in my heart. Something close to joy accompanied me into the cold room for the ultrasound. Barry and I were looking forward to sending the text, "Fifth year all clear!" to our family and going out to celebrate by eating dim sum. For five years, the scans had been negative and the blood work boded well.

So when the technician left and brought in the radiologist to review her findings, I remained unruffled, quietly awaiting the good news.

"Mrs. Chole," she began, "this is the second time I've had to say this today to someone who came in for their five-year check-in. I'm sad to say that the cancer has returned."

What? I thought. *But I had peace.*

Throughout the next two disillusioning years, Jesus and I did a lot of work together around my theology of peace. Ever since interrupting my life, Jesus had guided me into His will through the peace that came as I waited on Him and immersed myself in His Word.

In time, I realized that I had overextended my interpretation of that peace. Yes, it was how God led me, but no, it was not a foreshadowing of what God was leading me into.

I had peace because I had Jesus. He was with me and was leading me . . . straight into a desert.

I remember being greatly comforted at the time by an honest entry in Oswald Chambers's personal diary:

> There is an interesting puzzle in my mind concerning the intuitions born in communion with God. For instance, I had such a joyous confidence that the war would end this year, but there is no apparent likelihood that it will. It is just another indication of how little we dare trust anything but our Lord Himself. Again, there are intuitions born in the same way splendidly and wonderfully fulfilled. It makes it clear that the Holy Spirit must be recognized as the sagacious Ruler in all affairs and not our astute common sense.[2]

Well, I mused, *if Oswald Chambers can get it wrong, Alicia Britt Chole certainly can, too.*

Though grateful to have lost an illusion about the purpose of peace, another frustration still plagued me. The very thought of an upcoming scan would increase my heart rate and brim my eyes with tears. *Lord,* I pled, *this is ridiculous!* Then, again and again, I would speak truth to my soul.

> *This is scanxiety* [scan anxiety] *and it's a common experience among cancer patients. These emotions are more chemical than spiritual; my amygdala is "just doing its job."*[3] *Regardless of my feelings or the results, I know God will be with me and my family. I can only do what I can do and leave all of it with Him. Thankfully, it's always been caught early and my prognosis is quite good.*

True.

The words did calm the scanxiety (somewhat). But I still could not shake the sadness. I was so frustrated by my inability to tame my emotions with logic. Like the psalmist, I kept asking my soul why it was downcast when my hope was clearly in God.

Then one day, an image came to my mind in prayer. I saw a small pool of water kept in place by an encircling low mound of soil. The berm contained and tamed the water, preventing its overflow to nearby land. Processing the image, I sensed God's gentle instruction: *Alicia, like that little mound, your logic has been trying to tame and contain your grief. Let the berm down, my love. There is land beyond your logic that needs to be watered by your tears.*

And so, I wept—and have, on occasion, kept weeping—with confidence that my tears (and not just my mind) have an assignment in the midst of spiritual pain.

Perhaps the psalmist would have said to me, *Yes and amen.*

Chapter 28

...

SOMETHING NEW

New Testament evidence of disillusionment with self is also abundant. Throughout the Gospels, the disciples' illusions about their personal abilities, spiritual authority, and strength of devotion to Jesus collided with reality on a regular basis.

For example, in Matthew 16:16-17, Father God revealed to Peter that Jesus was "the Christ, the Son of the living God." In response to Peter's confession, Jesus spoke of building His church, and stated, "the gates of Hades will not overcome it. I will give you the keys of the kingdom of heaven; whatever you bind on earth will be bound in heaven, and whatever you loose on earth will be loosed in heaven" (Matthew 16:18-19). Which may have prompted Peter to think, *Keys of the kingdom? YESSSS!*

Immediately after this moment of revelation, Jesus began to speak of His soon-coming death more pointedly. When Peter boldly addressed Jesus' pessimistic outlook, Jesus rebuked him, saying, "Get behind me, Satan! You are a stumbling block to me" (Matthew 16:23).

Um, ouch. I guess I misunderstood my place?

Then Jesus took Peter, James, and John up to a high mountain where they witnessed the Transfiguration, in which "His face shone like the sun, and his clothes became as white as the light. Just then there appeared before them Moses and Elijah, talking with Jesus" (Matthew 17:2-3).

To which Peter might have wondered, *Well, I still have no clue what I did to mess up in the last chapter, but this is awesome!*

And then,

> When they came to the crowd, a man approached Jesus and knelt before him. "Lord, have mercy on my son," he said. "He has seizures and is suffering greatly. He often falls into the fire or into the water. I brought him to your disciples, but they could not heal him." . . . Jesus rebuked the demon, and it came out of the boy, and he was healed from that moment. Then the disciples came to Jesus in private and asked, "Why couldn't we drive it out?" He replied, "Because you have so little faith."
>
> MATTHEW 17:14-16, 18-20

What? I'm confused. Just a few verses ago You promised us that whatever we bound on earth would be bound in heaven. You don't lie. So what are we doing wrong?

This is the roller coaster of disillusionment inherent in applied faith. Armchair Christians have fewer challenges. But if we take God at His Word and step out in faith, odds are that we, like Peter and the early disciples, will lose a lot of sincere but inaccurate illusions about our abilities, our authority, and our devotion.

Thank God that almost all of these early leaders remained committed to their faith when disillusioned with themselves. With the exception of Judas, none of the Twelve bailed. But they sure came close!

The most well-known examples of disillusionment with self in the Gospels are recounted each Easter season. With admiration, we cheer at the disciples' courage when they each tell Jesus, "Even if I have to die with you, I will never disown you" (Matthew 26:35). Shocked, we shake our heads as Judas seals his betrayal with a kiss (see Matthew 26:48-49). Astonished, we watch as Jesus yields to arrest and "all the disciples deserted him and fled" (Matthew 26:56).

But when Peter denies all knowledge of Jesus three times, that rooster crows, and Jesus' and Peter's eyes meet (see Luke 22:54-61), we are gripped by something far more penetrating than admiration, shock, or astonishment. We are gripped by empathy. We are awakened to a shared, and sometimes horrifying, vulnerability. With Peter, we stand exposed and, disillusioned with our very selves, join him in weeping "bitterly" (Luke 22:62).

As I have written about elsewhere, "Peter wept because Peter loved. Peter's illusion was not that he loved Jesus. Peter's illusion was that he loved Jesus more than he loved his own life."[1] Getting things wrong is part of growing faith up. When we commit ourselves to love, revelations of lovelessness accompany us. As we lose illusions about our abilities, authority, and devotion, we gain greater understanding of God's acceptance, mercy, and grace. And our love—purified through the night—is strengthened.

Disillusionment with self occurs when assumptions about the life of faith collide with the frailty of our humanity, the persistence of our sins, the weakness of our wills, and the fact that transformation simply takes time. Such collisions humble us, sober us, and prepare the soil of our souls for true spiritual growth.

Have you ever made noble, heartfelt commitments, yet in the moment of testing denied the life of Christ within you? Have you ever been frustrated by weakness or stunned by failure?

Please remember that you are in good company. Along with King David (who experienced disillusionment with himself repeatedly), have you ever cried out, "Have mercy on me, O God, according to your unfailing love; according to your great compassion blot out my transgressions" (Psalm 51:1)?

In such times, when an earthquake reveals internal fault lines that you never knew existed—when the ground shakes beneath your feet and you fall into disillusionment with yourself—remember to get back up, receive forgiveness, and call upon your newly acquired humility to inspire others to commit to the way of love.[2]

Chapter 29

· · ·

CHASING HORSES

Oswald Chambers, in his teaching on the book of Job, explained,

> Intellect asks, "What is truth?" . . . as if truth were something
> that could be stated in words. "I am . . . the Truth," said Jesus
> (John 14:6). The only way we get at Truth is by life and person-
> ality. When a man is up against things it is no use for him to try
> and work it out logically, but let him obey, and instantly he will
> see his way through. Truth is moral, not intellectual. We perceive
> Truth by doing the right thing, not by thinking it out.[1]

Fascinating. This brilliant mind spoke of the limitations *of thinking* and
the strength *of doing* the "right thing" when we find ourselves in the
middle of a night. When disillusioned, our commitment to keep following Jesus—especially when we have no clue where He is leading—is more
powerful than we can imagine.

A long time ago, I came across quite a different story about another brilliant soul who faced a choice in the middle of a spiritual night. But before
sharing his journey, I need to set the stage with a story closer to home.

My family lives in the country with three dogs, two cats, and neighbors
that are cows. (I mean that in the nicest of ways. Our home is partially

surrounded by a dairy farm that features black-and-white classic cows.) Here in our quiet county, there are no leash laws, but somehow our dogs know their boundaries: this fence line, that dirt road, and the dry creek bed. They stay and play well within the safety of our few acres *except* when our other neighbor's horses draw near.

Then, our pups wander.

They cross under the wire to bark and run around and be a general nuisance to the horses, who maintain a sophisticated air of *We don't care* throughout the whole ordeal. I watch with both amusement and concern knowing that one of these days, our pups just might get the wind kicked out of them. Nonetheless, despite the danger, our dogs cannot seem to resist wandering when horses come into view.

Which has prompted me to think about how easy it is for us to wander in the presence of that one thing. What is it for us currently? What "horses" are we compelled to see up close and chase? What views invite us to step across lines of safety that have been established for our protection and take a risk for . . . well, for what? Perhaps for the thrill, the experience, the knowledge, the post-worthy story, or the rush?

Chasing horses.

Horses have been chased by many great thinkers, one of whom wrote a beautiful and inspiring hymn. In "Come, Thou Fount," Robert Robinson asked of God, "Let Thy goodness, like a fetter, bind my wandering heart to Thee." His prayer then spilled over into a captivating chorus:

> *Prone to wander, Lord, I feel it,*
> *Prone to leave the God I love;*
> *Here's my heart, O take and seal it;*
> *Seal it for Thy courts above.*[2]

Prone to wander. *O God, I feel it.*

Jerry Jenkins notes that Robinson[3] committed his life to Jesus from a "life of sin," wrote the hymn in 1757 in his early twenties, entered the ministry, became a preacher, and then "lapsed into sin again."[4]

In the years following the release of "Come, Thou Fount," Robinson became known as a respected thinker. Then, toward the end of his life,

> The story is told that Robinson was one day riding a stagecoach when he noticed a woman deeply engrossed with a hymn book. During an ensuing conversation the lady turned to Robinson and asked what he thought of the hymn she was humming. Robinson burst into tears and said, "Madam, I am the poor unhappy man who wrote that hymn many years ago, and I would give a thousand worlds, if I had them, to enjoy the feelings I had then."[5]

Robinson seems to have mourned what he lost through his wanderings.

Which brings me back home.

Though my dogs do not seem to be able to resist wandering, we *can*. But not in our own strength. This realization leads us to the first (of what will be eight) of my favorite tools for navigating this type of night.

WHEN DISILLUSIONED WITH YOURSELF, ASK GOD TO MENTOR YOUR MIND.

This is an intensely practical principle for me. We tend to think *about* God more than *with* God. Asking God to mentor our minds shifts the language in our thought life to more accurately reflect the truth that God is with us. So, instead of "Do *I* want to think about this right now?" we ask, "Jesus, do *we* want to think about this right now?"

Like many, I enjoy thinking, processing, and wrestling with thorny theological subjects. But sometimes I bump up against a fence post and sense the gentle whisper of God saying, "Let it rest for now. For the moment, no farther." And I have a choice to make. Will I press past that invisible barrier simply because I can? Or will I pause and trust the mentoring of the Holy Spirit whose entire purpose is to "guide [me] into all truth" (John 16:13)?

Sometimes—especially in academic environments, where it seems that if we *can* think about an issue, then we *must* think about an issue—I have, in the name of intellectual integrity, pressed past God's gentle whisper and entered territory that God knew well, but I was unprepared to navigate.[6]

With infinite patience, over many years, God has graciously shown me that true intellectual strength is not the ability to think. True intellectual strength is the ability *to choose* what to think and when to think.

Horses you want to chase today—subjects and concepts that you want to explore—may be easily ridden in years to come. As I said, the territory is familiar to your Master Mentor. But when you pursue such horses prematurely, odds are you are going to get the wind kicked out of you.

So, when disillusioned with yourself, ask God to mentor your mind. Ask Him to lead your thoughts with a prayer, something like this:

> *Lord,*
> *at this time,*
> *do I have Your permission*
> *to go here in my thoughts*
> *with You?*

(Frankly, if I cannot go somewhere *with* Him, I really do not want to wander there *without* Him.)

As Robinson wrote so long ago, "Let Thy goodness, like a fetter, bind my wandering heart to Thee."

Chapter 30

. . .

HEART MATTERS

Between our kitchen and living room is a smudged, smeared doorframe in desperate need of a fresh coat of paint. But I cannot (and probably will not) ever pick up a brush because the frame is etched with glorious lines, names, and dates marking measurements of my kids growing up. In my memory, I still see them standing as tall as they can with the best posture of the day (or year) and lifting their heads high to get every centimeter possible.

Physical growth is visible, tangible, quantifiable, and (for the most part) indisputable. We celebrate this kind of growth and mark it on the doorways of our lives. But what of other kinds of growth? To the point, how do we measure, how do we monitor, how do we celebrate growth that is *within*?

If we were to pose this question to church attenders, we might hear responses like "I know I'm spiritually growing when . . ."

God's blessing is obvious. *(I'm prosperous.)*

Things I put my hand to go well. *(Life is easier.)*

I've earned the good opinion of good people. *(I'm established.)*

I'm taking new territory and reaping the rewards. *(My influence is growing, and I'm bearing fruit.)*

I talk about my faith freely. *(God is on my lips.)*

We tend to look at these outward *signs* and retroactively attribute inward growth to ourselves. In other words, "Look at all this. I must be doing something right."

Maybe.

I wonder if the prophet Jeremiah might say, "Maybe not."

Consider, once again, one of my favorite complaints in the Scriptures:

> You are always righteous, O LORD,
>   when I bring a case before you.
> Yet I would speak with you about your justice:
>   Why does the way of the wicked *prosper?*
>   Why do all the faithless *live at ease?*
> You have planted them, and *they have taken root;*
>   they *grow and bear fruit.*
> You are always *on their lips*
>   but far from their hearts.[1]
> JEREMIAH 12:1-2, EMPHASIS ADDED

Evidently, prosperity, ease, stability, success, and religious speech are not absolute indicators of spiritual growth. Spiritual growth is a matter of the heart.

WHEN DISILLUSIONED WITH YOURSELF,
MAKE SURE YOUR SIGNS FOR SPIRITUAL GROWTH
ARE SPIRITUAL.

Especially if we have known privilege, we must be vigilant to avoid confusing abundance for obedience or social success for the favor of God. Yes, sometimes these pair powerfully hand in hand. However, throughout the ages, the saints who have gone before us affirm that the greatest times of spiritual growth often take place in the darkest nights of life, when we are not visibly prospering, tangibly fruitful, relationally stable, or emotionally at ease.

Job's comforters would disagree. They sat for seven days in silence to honor Job's suffering, and then Eliphaz verbalized what they all assumed was obvious:

> "Who, being innocent, has ever perished? Where were the
> upright ever destroyed?"
> JOB 4:7

> "Is it for your piety that he rebukes you and brings charges
> against you? Is not your wickedness great? Are not your sins
> endless?"
> JOB 22:4-5

> "That is why snares are all around you, why sudden peril terrifies
> you, why it is so dark you cannot see, and why a flood of water
> covers you."
> JOB 22:10-11

In other words, "Job, bad things only happen to bad people."

In some ways, it would be simpler if this were true—if our circumstances were determined by our love for God. Then, only the spiritually healthy would become financially wealthy. Only those with purity would bear the burden of popularity. However, as Jesus said in His teaching on loving our enemies, "Your Father in Heaven . . . causes his sun to rise on the evil and the good, and sends rain on the righteous and the unrighteous" (Matthew 5:45).

So, if prosperity, ease, success, stability, and religious speech are not always indicators of spiritual growth, and if lack, difficulty, failure, uncertainty, and everyday speech are not always indicators of spiritual decline, how then do we know when we are spiritually growing?

The word *grow* appears in various forms over 130 times in my study Bible.[2] It is translated from dozens of Hebrew, Aramaic, and Greek words, all of which carry meanings related to *increase, multiplication,* and *growth.* Since no single word in the Old or New Testaments captures a significant percentage of those occurrences, I studied each appearance in a search for biblical signs of spiritual growth.

In the Old Testament, *grow* is most often used in the realm of agriculture (e.g., the growth of trees, grains, flocks, herds), physical and emotional human development (e.g., growing up, old, strong, weak, wise, faint), and finance (e.g., growing wealthy or poor).

In the New Testament, however, over half of the twenty-three occur-rences[3] relate to some form of spiritual growth, while the rest reference agriculture (e.g., the growth of flowers, wheat, mustard seeds) or physical and emotional human development (e.g., growing up, weary, bitter). I will leave the study to you,[4] but, in summary, the New Testament writers encouraged the early church to grow in

knowledge of and love for God,

appreciation for salvation,

gratitude for grace, and

godly love for others.

So, where might we look for evidence, *biblically,* of spiritual growth? In whether we are . . .

losing illusions and gaining reality about God and His love, increasingly aware of what we were saved from and for,

more and more thankful for God's generosity to us as sinners, and

trying to show others the love God has shown to us.

In other words, disillusionment, humility, thankfulness, and applied love are all signs of spiritual growth!

I think (well, I hope) that Jeremiah would agree.

Chapter 31

...

THAT SAME
OLD SPOT

If our definition of spiritual growth is not spiritual, we tend to prematurely attribute growth to ourselves in good times and unnecessarily be disillusioned with ourselves in difficult times. But even when we make the shift and begin evaluating spiritual growth based on internal movements instead of external circumstances, progress can still be a mystery to us, particularly when it seems that the path is taking us backward instead of forward.

And yes, it is possible to go backward.

If we keep caressing things that Jesus was crucified for, we will move backward by choice. If we willfully continue in behaviors and interactions that Jesus named when taking upon Himself the sins of the world, we will lose spiritual ground. As Oswald Chambers taught, "Deliverance from sin is not deliverance from human nature. There are things in our human nature which must be destroyed by neglect; there are other things which must be destroyed by active attack, that is by the Divine strength imparted by God's Spirit."[1]

The context of this next principle, however, is not willful disobedience but rather those times in life when, while trying to follow Jesus, we keep passing that same old spot: *There it is again. I thought I was past this, but evidently not.*

WHEN DISILLUSIONED WITH YOURSELF,
TRADE IN YOUR LINE FOR A SPIRAL.

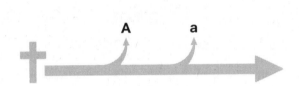

Many inherit a view of spiritual growth that is linear. New life begins as we commit ourselves to Jesus. For some, like myself, that moment is distinct. For others, particularly those who grew up in church, that moment may be more like waking up: though difficult to isolate the exact second we awoke, there came a point in time when we knew, beyond a shadow of a doubt, that we were no longer sleeping.

From this starting point, when we view spiritual growth as a straight line, we anticipate that there will be challenges, but we expect to see each one *only once*. For example, perhaps early on in our faith walk, God convicts us of unforgiveness toward a parent. In response, we pause, repent, ask forgiveness, rise forgiven, and keep moving, fully expecting never to deal with that issue again. So, when it pops back up a few years later—maybe after a painful interaction with a leader or the opportunity to become a parent ourselves—we can become quite confused.

Wait a minute, I already addressed this way back there.

But maybe I wasn't really repentant then.

Or perhaps, for some reason, God didn't hear or forgive me.

Could it be that He didn't hear me because I don't really know Him?

If this sounds familiar, I have some really good news: forgiveness is dependent upon Jesus' sacrificial offering, not our perfect asking. Sincere repentance is most certainly heard by the God who knows and loves us fully. The real problem is that a linear view of spiritual growth is not complex enough for a genuine life of faith.

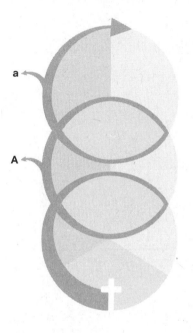

Instead of a straight line, think of spiritual growth as a three-dimensional spiral. Unlike a thin line (that seems all too easy to fall off), spiritual growth is more like an upward winding path in which we do revisit issues but on different levels. That same old spot is not in the same old place. Addressing an old issue in a new season is often a sign of growth, not of failure. Because we *do* know God, because He *does* hear and forgive us, because our repentance *was* sincere, we are now poised for God to attend to that old weakness at the next level in our souls.

This truth became more vivid to me through a minor surgery. My dad was a golfer back in the day when golfers wore crazy, wild, bold pants and shirts. The only thing brighter than Dad's clothes on the course when he played was his face. He maintained a season-round sunburn and, not surprisingly, contracted skin cancer later in life. Around the same time, a dermatologist found a spot of skin cancer on me, which meant that we both had surgeries within a year of each other. Dad's experience, however, was entirely different from mine.

My dermatologist numbed up the area nicely, sliced off the skin cancer gingerly, sewed me up quickly, revived me with orange juice, and I was on my way within the hour.

My dad's surgery was an ordeal. After the dermatologist sliced off a layer of skin, he had Dad wait while the sample was biopsied. Then, in an hour or so, the dermatologist returned, sliced off another layer, and Dad waited once again for the biopsy. This process repeated itself the entire day until finally, the doctor had a sample that was cancer-free (and Dad had a deep gash above his cheekbone).

Occasionally, spiritual growth is more like my surgery.

> God reveals an issue.
>
> We attend to the issue.
>
> We rise renewed and/or forgiven regarding the issue.
>
> And we never see that issue again for the rest of our lives.

However, as has been true in my own journey, spiritual growth is more often like my dad's surgery.

> God reveals an issue.
>
> We attend to the issue.
>
> We rise renewed and/or forgiven regarding the issue.
>
> And (thank Him), He lets us rest.
>
> Then, later on, further up the spiral, God addresses that issue *again*—accessing the next layer needed for health in our souls.

This is advance, not retreat. This is growth, not failure. This is God revisiting vulnerable areas as often as needed in His commitment to eradicate all spiritual cancer within us.

So, when disillusioned with yourself, remember: apart from willful disobedience, often the reason we see the same issue again and again is because *we are growing.* As Paul said, "Now the Lord is the Spirit, and where the Spirit of the Lord is, there is freedom. And we, who with unveiled faces all reflect the Lord's glory, are being transformed into his likeness with ever-increasing glory, which comes from the Lord, who is the Spirit" (2 Corinthians 3:17-18).

Or, to quote the words of an old song from an unknown author:

From glory to glory He's changing me,
Changing me, changing me;
His likeness and image to perfect in me,
The love of God shown to the world.[2]

Chapter 32

. . .

GAINING GROUND

The word is old and rather rare.[1] But it captures an agonizing reality that is common to all. As an adjective, *besetting* first appeared in 1796 in *Joan of Arc: An Epic Poem* written by Robert Southey.[2] The word described sin—specifically the type of sin referenced in Hebrews 12:1: "Therefore, since we are surrounded by such a great cloud of witnesses, let us throw off everything that hinders and the sin that so easily entangles, and let us run with perseverance the race marked out for us."

The sin that so easily entangles. This is what *besetting* means. As a verb, *beset* is defined as "to set or station themselves around, to surround with hostile intent; to set upon or assail on all sides; to besiege."[3] Perhaps all of us are acquainted with this type of sin.

Distinct from willful disobedience (when *we want* to sin), this is sin we feel pursued by (as though *it wants us*). We long to be free of it but keep falling into it. Being quick to anger, bingeing, self-medicating, critical or controlling behaviors, addictions, impurity, revisionism, pride, greed—the list is long. And the experience is not new.

I find this law at work: When I want to do good, evil is right there with me. For in my inner being I delight in God's law; but I see another law at work in the members of my body, waging war against the law of my mind and making me a prisoner of the law of sin at work within my members. What a wretched man I am! Who will rescue me from this body of death? Thanks be to God—through Jesus Christ our Lord!

ROMANS 7:21-25

There is war going on, both around us and within us. Sadly, since the Fall, sin seeds are indigenous to our souls. Gladly, since the Cross, Jesus has defeated sin and death.

Along the way, however, our struggle with besetting sins can be very disillusioning. We read that "in all these things we are more than conquerors through him who loved us" (Romans 8:37) and wonder why we still feel like losers. In *context*, this verse is sandwiched between Paul's inspiring treatise on how nothing can separate us from God's love. In the *moment*, however, we just feel woefully unworthy of anyone's love.

Besetting sins often have deep (sometimes generations-deep) roots or origins involving trauma. Though the principle I am about to offer is in no way a substitute for the hard work of biblical counseling and self-discipline, it has helped many gain ground in the battle.

WHEN DISILLUSIONED WITH YOURSELF, CRITIQUE YOUR DEFINITION OF VICTORY.

"It's hopeless," he said. "I think it's behind me, but then I fall into sin again. No matter what I do, this thing will not let go."

His fight had been long. Joe (obviously not his real name) had struggled with impurity since childhood. For weeks, and even months, he would resist temptation, but then fall back into the same old sins.

Each time the pit got a little deeper.

Each time his hope got a little dimmer.

Now, as an adult, he had tried everything he knew to break the cycle: repentance, accountability, Bible study, Scripture memorization, therapy, prayer counseling, and fasting. Utterly disillusioned with his ability to obey God, he wept and said, "I will never have victory in this area."

While my husband listened to him attentively, I sat nearby, praying while they interacted. Over and over, a question kept coming to mind, and I knew it needed to be asked.

"Joe," I began, "you keep saying that you will never have victory in this area. What would victory look like to you?"

"That's easy," he replied. "Victory is the day I wake up and no longer *want* to sin."

For decades, this dear man had believed that the desire to sin *was* sin— that being attracted to impurity meant he had already been defeated by impurity. His definition of victory was the absence of *want to*, not the presence of *will to*.

Victory sourced in feelings is not viable.

Our feelings can be affected by everything from allergy-season sadness to sunshine-stimulated serotonin. Defining a word as weighty as *victory* through the presence or absence of something as flighty as feelings will continually place victory out of our reach.

The *Oxford English Dictionary*'s first two definitions of *victory* are as follows:

1. The position or state of having overcome an enemy or adversary in combat, battle, or war.
2. An instance or occasion of overcoming an adversary in battle, etc.; a triumph gained by force of arms.[4]

Not only is victory the stuff of choices (not feelings), victory can be validly celebrated each "instance or occasion" of action, not just after the entire war has been won.

For example, consider a young woman struggling with an eating disorder. Regardless of how low the number on the scale goes, she looks in the mirror and still sees herself as "fat." Is victory for this soul postponed until a day when she looks in the mirror and no longer *feels* fat? Granted, that would be a wonderful day, but victory can be valid much, much earlier. Victory can be celebrated each time she looks in the mirror, still feels fat, and thinks, *But those whom I trust say it is not true. God, help me today to honor You by taking a step to take care of my body.* That is victory! Not because her emotions have politely surrendered themselves to truth, but because she is exercising her will to choose life.

Or consider a very different kind of struggle in the Garden of Gethsemane. There, Jesus "began to be deeply distressed and troubled" (Mark 14:33), and said, "My soul is overwhelmed with sorrow to the point of death" (Matthew 26:38). Alone in prayer, He pleaded, "*Abba*, Father . . . everything is possible for you. Take this cup from me" (Mark 14:36). "And being in anguish, he prayed more earnestly, and his sweat was like drops of blood falling to the ground" (Luke 22:44).

In the realm of emotions, were Jesus' feelings in Gethsemane a reflection of His Father's will? Was He filled with joy and excitement at the prospect of taking the sins of the world upon Himself through the cross?

Clearly not.

In fact, He even asked for the cup to pass if possible.

In that dreadful night, Jesus' emotions were not in sync with the Father's will for Him. So, did Jesus sin? Did Jesus fail? No and no. Jesus was victorious. Not because He lacked uncooperative feelings, but because He *chose to obey*. Jesus' "Yet not what I will, but what you will!" (Mark 14:36) shook the earth with the sound of victory, and yours can too!

Our generation is being held back by the fallacy that *doing* something without first *feeling* something is hypocritical. Like Joe, we sit disillusioned with ourselves needlessly, waiting for our feelings to change in order for us to declare victory.

Thankfully, with or without the cooperation of our emotions, our wills can be exercised to keep following Jesus all the way to and through every night.

As a postscript, you might be interested to know that Joe did overcome. Is he still vulnerable? Of course. Vulnerable and victorious.

Chapter 33

...

NEVER WASTED

One of the most alarming aspects of disillusionment with self is the vulnerability we feel in the midst of it. Seeing ourselves more accurately is humbling. Not being as strong—or wise, or mature, or loving—as we thought we were is sobering. Though we are grateful that God's "power is made perfect in [our] weakness" (2 Corinthians 12:9), we would prefer to not be weak at all.

This frequently referenced verse was penned by Paul in his plea for God to remove a "thorn in [his] flesh" (2 Corinthians 12:7). To Paul's distress, the thorn remained, as has endless speculation as to what the thorn actually was. Could it have been persecution, oppression, annoyance, loss of sight, malaria, temptation, or migraines? Opinions are abundant, but evidence is lacking that would lead us to any certainty.

Of this, however, we can be sure: by God's description, it was a weakness—one in which God promised to make His power known.

WHEN DISILLUSIONED WITH YOURSELF,
LISTEN TO WHAT GOD WHISPERS THROUGH WEAKNESS.

In the realm of faith, weakness is never wasted. In fact, God has a history of whispering to His people when they feel weak. Among the more well-known examples is the story we considered earlier, when Elijah ran for his life in fear of Jezebel. After cycles of sleeping and eating, Elijah reached Horeb and went into a cave. When God told him to go stand on the mountain because He was about to pass by,

> a great and powerful wind tore the mountains apart and shattered the rocks before the LORD, but the LORD was not in the wind. After the wind there was an earthquake, but the LORD was not in the earthquake. After the earthquake came a fire, but the LORD was not in the fire. And after the fire came a gentle whisper. When Elijah heard it, he pulled his cloak over his face and went out and stood at the mouth of the cave.
>
> 1 KINGS 19:11-13

When Elijah felt like a failure and was disillusioned with himself to the point of despair, God came to him—not in the power of wind, earthquake, or fire, but in a gentle whisper.

God still whispers to us in our weakness. Wisdom invites us to listen. As with Elijah, God's voice when we are weak is often *directional*.

One wise father, when asked how his child's diagnosis with autism had changed his life, described his son as "my built-in Sabbath."[1] In no way was he implying that life was calm, but rather that his personal pace had slowed. His son's needs had reshaped and redirected his life. Many have discovered a more sustainable rhythm through God's whispers in what the world calls weakness.

Still, our resistance to weakness is understandable. Surely most would prefer to be strong mentally, emotionally, physically, and relationally. Weakness changes our plans, edits our dreams, and, perhaps even more challenging, affects those around us.

I remember a conversation long ago with a vulnerable soul who confessed, "I don't want to be the weak link. I don't want to be what holds my husband back." She had tried desperately to power through, not wanting to hinder her husband's potential, until the day when her body collapsed. In the subsequent crisis, instead of running the race together, they both stood still as God's whispers guided them into unforeseen paths and an even deeper love for one another. Her devoted husband stood still with her, and together, they listened as God's whisper guided them into unforeseen paths and an even deeper love for one another.

God whispered to me in my weakness in an unexpected way many years ago. One morning, I woke up and noticed tiny red dots on my finger. *That's odd*, I thought, and went on with my day. Soon the red dots became tender, and it dawned on me that somehow a set of splinters had made their way into my finger. I had not noticed, but my body did. Its natural healing properties had been pushing the splinters to the surface.

My view, however, only got worse. The dots became angry as the splinters worked their way out. Of course, I could have resisted and pressed them back down. But why would anyone resist healing? In time, the splinters all came out, the tenderness subsided, the dots remained for a season, and eventually all visible signs of the event were gone.

The timing of this experience was a gift. As a young missionary serving university students in another land, I was thrilled by all that God was doing on the campus and disillusioned by what was happening within myself. I was struggling with an area of sin and frustrated by my slow progress. Until God sent me encouragement through this set of splinters.

I have never heard God's voice audibly, though there have been a few times in my life in which His voice within was so loud, I thought others could surely hear it. Personally, God "speaks to me" as I open His Word and still myself before Him. I will attempt to paraphrase what I felt God whispering to me that day when, disillusioned with myself, I dissolved in a puddle of tears.

Daughter, remember the splinters. Before you saw your sin, I saw your sin. Before you had any idea that something needed attention, My Spirit was already pushing the area to the surface. The only reason you can see it now, child, is that, by My grace, it's on its way out.

What a relief.

God does not show us our weakness to mock us. God reveals to heal.

In between revelation and healing, things may look worse before they get better (especially if we resist the revelation or keep pushing the problem back into our lives). But like those splinters, the only reason we can see the issue now is that, by God's Spirit, it is on its way out!

We tend to want the process to be instantaneous. But as we wait, we can be encouraged that "He who began a good work in you, will carry it onto completion until the day of Christ Jesus" (Philippians 1:6).

A day *will* come when "He will wipe every tear from [our] eyes. There will be no more death or mourning or crying or pain" (Revelation 21:4). Until then, when disillusioned with ourselves, let us lean in to listen for God's whispers, knowing that somehow, His "power is made perfect in [our] weakness" (2 Corinthians 12:9).

Chapter 34

. . .

FILTERING
"FAILURES"

The word *failure* can haunt us when we are disillusioned with ourselves. Phrases like *I'm such a failure* can weigh our souls down to the point of despair. Though failure is possible, it seems to me that we have overstretched its definition and, consequently, its application.

Not everyone struggles with this, but those who do understand how exhausting it is to live under an overly broad definition of failure that includes everything short of perfection. How we define failure matters because what we say to ourselves when disillusioned is formative.

Accuracy strengthens us.

Inaccuracy does not.

WHEN DISILLUSIONED WITH YOURSELF,
REMEMBER THAT NOT ALL FAILURE IS SIN.

Early in my faith walk, a campus leader's generosity helped me experience this distinction firsthand. As a new follower of Jesus, I had roughly a thousand ideas of how my university ministry could share Jesus with others. One proposal, however, stood out among all the others. I was sure it was *the key* to bringing hundreds of college students to Christ.

"We'll hold an evangelistic aerobics outreach!" I beamed.

The campus pastor blinked a few times and then said, "Go on."

So, on I went, gushing about plans to gather prayer requests at the end of each workout, preparations to visit those who came to exercise, and potential promotional materials. The leader said what many leaders would say to me in the years to come: "Alicia, that's an idea." Then he added, "Why don't you go do that? Have a good time."

Off I went to reserve a space, design a worthy workout, canvass the campus with invites, and pray my little heart out in anticipation of the many souls about to meet Jesus. But when the day finally came, no one else did. As in *ever*. For the entire six-session outreach, it was just me, my music, and a bunch of lonely floor mats.

Was my evangelistic aerobics outreach a failure? Yes. Perhaps the simplest definition of failure is "a lack of success."[1] Since the event's entire purpose was to gather students who might be open to learning more about Jesus and no one ever came, this qualified.

However, did Jesus die on the cross *to forgive me* for holding an evangelistic aerobics outreach?

No.

Not at all.

Because not all failure is sin.

In fact, failure is one of the wisest teachers in the growth process (if we let it speak).

Looking back, surely something successful would have been better for the ministry's image. I will always be grateful that it was more important to the leadership for me to have the opportunity to learn that "failure was not fatal."[2] Though the outreach was a failure, I was not.

Which brings up a valid question: How do we know when a failure is simply part of the learning process and when a failure is sin?

In the New Testament, *fail* and its variations appear sixteen times in my study Bible, most famously in what is often referred to as the love chapter: "Love never fails" (1 Corinthians 13:8). However, only a few of these occurrences directly reference faith failures:

> [Jesus asked,] "Are your hearts hardened? Do you have eyes but fail to see, and ears but fail to hear? And don't you remember?"
> MARK 8:17-18

> [Jesus said,] "Simon, Simon, Satan has asked to sift you as wheat. But I have prayed for you, Simon, that your faith may not fail."
> LUKE 22:31-32

> We are weak in him, yet by God's power we will live with him to serve you. Examine yourselves to see whether you are in the faith; test yourselves. Do you not realize that Christ Jesus is in you—unless, of course, you fail the test? And I trust that you will discover that we have not failed the test.
> 2 CORINTHIANS 13:4-6

Obviously, the scriptural treatment of spiritual failure is not limited to appearances of the exact term. But these mentions in Jesus' and Paul's teachings can enlighten us. Jesus prayed that the faith of His followers would not fail. Then and now, such failure, from God's perspective, has to do with the hardening of a heart. And one of the paths to that hardening is through an untested, unexamined faith.

This is why I believe we need to be more careful in our use of the word *failure*. A hard heart is a serious thing, and the words we speak to ourselves are powerful. So, the next time you hear, *I'm such a failure* in your self-talk, for the sake of your future, please pause and do some evaluation. Ask yourself:

Did Jesus die for this?

Did I do this in disobedience?

Did I numb myself to or simply ignore the conviction of the Spirit?

If your answer is no, take a deep breath and refuse to confuse the failure with sin. If your answer is *yes*—if your spiritual failure is actual (as opposed to imagined against the backdrop of perfectionism or comparison), if you realize that Jesus *did* die on the cross for this—then repent. Ask His forgiveness *and forgive yourself.*

In other words, respect the reality that Jesus was already beaten up enough for the both of you.

Jesus' work on the cross was sufficient. It does God no honor—and yourself no good—to act as though there is more that needs to be paid. Receive Jesus' forgiveness. Rise forgiven. Surrender to the upward pull of God's love with renewed gratitude for His grace.

In life, when facing a perceived spiritual failure, four possibilities exist for your consideration.

First, it is not really a failure at all, but rather an unmet, unrealistic expectation of yourself. If so, take a closer look at Jesus and ask Him to help you make peace with your humanity.

Second, it is a failure, but not a sin. If so, view the failure as an unexpected teacher and learn from—but do not lament—the experience.

Third, it is a failure and a sin. If so, be thankful for tangible symptoms of sin's sickness. Confess your sins to God. Remember that, since He never had any illusions about you, His great love for you is as strong as it ever has been.

Fourth, the situation feels fuzzy, and you honestly cannot discern whether it is failure, a sin, or both. If so, wait in prayer. Ask God to speak to you with full assurance that, if sin is present, He will be faithful to reveal it.

Chapter 35

. . .

PICKLE SOUP

Perhaps some of the art in the Church has inadvertently contributed to why it can be difficult for us to distinguish between healthy learning, innocent failing, and willful sinning. Our depictions *of* Jesus can affect our understanding of what it means *to be like* Jesus.

For example, in our home is a painting of Jesus in the Garden of Gethsemane that has been a source of inspiration and peace for generations of my husband's family. Artistically, it is truly beautiful. But theologically, I find it curious. In the painting, Jesus is kneeling (with perfect posture), utterly serene (bathed in the warmth of his backlit, combed hair), with hands (that have never seen a day of work) gently folded in prayer (over a radiant rock).

I would never want to discount the real comfort this image has brought to others, but this depiction does not comfort me. This is not what descriptions like "sorrowful and troubled" (Matthew 26:37), "deeply distressed" (Mark 14:33), or "in anguish . . . and his sweat was like drops of blood" (Luke 22:44) inspire in my imagination.

Another example is probably much more familiar. As someone who did not grow up reading the Bible, one of my first impressions of how the

Church viewed their Jesus came through Christmas carols like "Away in a Manger" that portrayed baby Jesus with the phrase "no crying He makes." Hearing the lyrics as a young atheist, I remember thinking, *So, Jesus was so holy that he did not . . . cry?*

In Nativity plays, I understand why parents (and producers) soothe and quiet the baby standing in for Jesus, but perhaps a wailing infant actor might be more accurate? Surely baby Jesus bawled. Crying is not a sin. And surely Jesus looked like an agonized mess in Gethsemane the night He was betrayed. Feeling sorrowful is not a sin. Why then do our depictions sometimes tidy Him up?

The Incarnation is defined as the "central Christian doctrine that God became flesh, that God assumed a human nature and became a man in the form of Jesus Christ, the Son of God and the second person of the Trinity. Christ was truly God and truly man."[1]

We want to be like Jesus, but our understanding of what Jesus is like may be in need of repair. Instead of "truly God and truly man," perhaps our definition of the Incarnation is more often mostly God with a dash of man.

Since a skewed view of Jesus can actually contribute to the pressure we feel to be superhuman, consider your honest responses to the following:

> Imagine baby Jesus taking His first step. Do you see Him teetering and falling or standing the first time (and being selected for the Olympics shortly afterward)?

> Imagine Jesus attending a school that may have been connected to the local synagogue. Do you think He had the highest grades in the class? Is it conceivable that He might have had something less than an A in math?

> Imagine a track team at this hypothetical school. Do you assume that Jesus would have been the fastest? Could someone else have been the captain of the team?

Imagine Jesus crafting a bench in Joseph's shop. Do you think His first work was His best work? Is it possible that He had to scrap it and try again?

Personally, I imagine Jesus and Joseph smiling and laughing as together they dismantled Jesus' less-than-benchy first (and even fifth) bench.

Why?

Because Jesus did not come from heaven to earth to die for our growth curves.

Though we are all sinful, being human is not a sin. Jesus was human *and* holy. And the ideas we have surrounding these two attributes directly affect how we respond when disillusioned with ourselves.

Do we view tears as a lack of holiness? Do we believe that deep sorrow can coexist with great faith? Do our first efforts have to double as our all-time-best offerings?

In other words, do we give ourselves permission *to be human and grow?*

WHEN DISILLUSIONED WITH YOURSELF,
GIVE YOURSELF GRACE TO BE GROWING.

Two of the few verses that open a window into Jesus' hidden years describe Him with a magnificently human trait that it would serve us well to prize more generously:

And the child grew and became strong; he was filled with wisdom, and the grace of God was upon him.
LUKE 2:40

And Jesus grew in wisdom and stature, and in favor with God
and men.
LUKE 2:52

Jesus *grew*. He grew physically (in stature), relationally (in favor with
men), and spiritually (in wisdom and in favor with God).[2] Growing is not
failure. Growing means that we are more today than we were yesterday. If
this was true of Jesus, surely it can be true of us.

Surely God delights in (as opposed to merely tolerates) our growth just
as we delight in the growth of a child, which brings me to one of my
favorite memories.

"Here, Mama, taste this. I made it just for you!"

My daughter has always loved to cook. She inherited that passion from
my mom, whose primary love languages were giving gifts and feeding
people. Some of my most precious photos are of Granny and Keona side
by side, kneading and rolling out homemade tortillas in Granny's kitchen.
Fresh off the griddle with salted butter—oh my! Keona now carries on
the tradition like a pro.

Ever since she could reach the stove, Keona was experimenting in the
kitchen and making treats for us. Early on, her favorite fare was soup. I
would heat up a pot of water on the stove and she would fill it with all
things pretty: green pickles, red apples, yellow cheese, and pink cupcake
sprinkles. Blending all the ingredients together with supersecret season-
ings like mustard and salsa, Keona would signal me when her creation
was done and watch me with anticipation as I prepared to sample her gift.

A long time ago, I made a commitment to never lie to my kids. So, every
time while Keona looked on beaming, awaiting my response, I would sip
my soup and say, "Oh Keo, thank you! This is really something special!"

And it was. If not always to my taste buds, her offerings were always special to my heart. Keona's intent was to bless me, and that was enough. In fact, that was a treasure. She made a loving guess as to what would please me, and guess what? I felt both loved and pleased. Outside reviews of her soups were irrelevant. Regardless of what wonder she served me, her heart was the ingredient that brought me joy.

Allow me to pose what will initially seem to be a ridiculous question: Were Keona's pickley, sprinkley, cheesy culinary inventions *unsuccessful*? Should these early efforts have disillusioned her? Embarrassed her? Called into question her potential as an aspiring chef?

Of course not.

Keona and I were spending time together doing something she enjoyed. She loved me and was using her creativity to offer me a gift. From my perspective, this was about as far away from unsuccessful as she could possibly get.

Deeming such efforts *unsuccessful* would make no sense at all, **unless** your definition of *success* is . . .

> never giving the critics any fodder for criticism,
>
> meeting or exceeding everyone's highest expectations,
>
> starting at the same level of excellence with which you hope to end, or
>
> not in need of instruction or correction to achieve further growth.

How often is disillusionment *with* ourselves inspired by unrealistic expectations *of* ourselves? And how often are our expectations shaped not by our God, but by our anxiety, fear of rejection, perfectionism, pursuit of favor, or tendency to measure ourselves comparatively?

Yes, growing can be uncomfortable and even embarrassing. But theologically, growing should not be shaming.

Therefore, the next time you are disillusioned with yourself, pause long enough to prayerfully identify what is *really* troubling you. If it is not sin, then what is it? Sometimes we are disillusioned with ourselves not because we are losing illusions and gaining reality (which is healthy), but because we have not given ourselves permission *to be human* (which is unsustainable). You are allowed (and even encouraged) to be human. Look past the disgrace and consider God's proud-parent face. See Him with you, celebrating your stumbling steps just as you would celebrate the growth of a beloved child.

All who breathe are in process.

May God help us cease villainizing our humanity.

Grow with grace and freedom, my friend! Make your soups with love. Fill them with pickles, and cheese, and apples, and sprinkles. Your Savior will think they are wonderful! (And in truth, His is the only palate we need to please.)

Chapter 36

. . .

THE COMMON
THREAD

These principles for navigating disillusionment with self all share a common thread: grace. Of grace, psychologist Lewis Smedes said the following:

> Grace overcomes shame, not by uncovering an overlooked cache of excellence in ourselves but simply by accepting us, the whole of us, with no regard to our beauty or our ugliness, our virtue or our vices. We are accepted wholesale. . . . Accepted once and accepted forever. Accepted at the ultimate depth of our being.[1]

> Many of us feel shame not for our too-badness but for our not-good-enoughness.[2]

> Grace heals our shame . . . by removing the one thing all our shame makes us fear the most: rejection.[3]

Grace appears 131 times in my study Bible, with 94 percent of occurrences in the New Testament. The early church understood *the grace of God* to be a benefactor like no other. In their greetings and benedictions, they prayed for God's grace to accompany, guide, gift, and guard one another.

One Greek word, *charis*, accounts for all New Testament occurrences of the word "grace." Books and writings abound on this almost inconceivable concept. As one study guide noted, "**Grace** in simple terms is God's unmerited favor and supernatural enablement and empowerment for salvation and for daily sanctification. *Grace is everything for nothing to those who don't deserve anything.* Grace is what every man needs, what none can earn and what God Alone can and does freely give."[4]

Grace (God's unmerited favor) must be stewarded with integrity. Though God's grace is immutable, we are fully capable of misapplication. Ours is a generation that celebrates living by the golden rule, just without the "rule" part. We treasure God's promise of "My grace is sufficient for you" (2 Corinthians 12:9), but we sometimes overlook the verse's context. God's sufficient grace was for Paul's unspecified and unwanted weakness, not for lawlessness masquerading as liberty.

An anything-goes religion tends to abuse the gift of grace.

But overcompensating—expecting too much of ourselves in order to avoid expecting too little of ourselves—misses grace as well.

Overcompensating is an exercise in futility. It hurts us and helps no one. One soul being unhealthy has never helped another soul find health.

I am aware that the phrase "expecting too much of ourselves" may be grating. One might ask, "How can we possibly expect too much of ourselves after Christ has given His all for us?" By not giving ourselves (or others) the freedom to fail in whatever their rendition of an *evangelistic aerobics outreach* might be. By demanding that our *first soups* be worthy of Michelin stars. By delaying *true victory* through defining it emotionally or refusing to forgive ourselves even though Christ (at great cost) has already pronounced us forgiven. In short, by forgetting

that we are human,

that growth is a given for humanity,

and that Jesus died for our sins, not for our growth curves.

Grace is the key. And grace is what makes my next encouragement possible.

WHEN DISILLUSIONED WITH YOURSELF, VIEW FAITH AS A PILGRIMAGE INSTEAD OF A PERFORMANCE.

The timing escapes me. In fact, much of the entire process escapes me. It felt like waking up from a surgery, clueless as to the intricacies of the operation but immediately benefiting from the surgeons' good work. My only contribution had been to trust the professionals and stay still under the knife.

Mixing (or rather shifting) metaphors, one day I realized that God had been conducting guerilla warfare within my soul. Beneath my barely begun new life of faith, a quiet coup d'état was occurring. Generaled by God's Spirit, in skirmishes too deep for observation, *fear was being deposed* and *love was being enthroned* as the ruling motivator in my life.

Over the years, that overthrow has been both gradual and continual. Almost every time I enter a new season in life, I have to reconfirm that love, not fear, will take the lead.

Why? Because alliances with fear are all too easy to make, especially in the night.

Fear disguises itself as *realism*, and we invite it to the table.

Fear presents itself as *troubleshooting*, and we welcome its wisdom.

Fear offers itself as a *prophet*, and we sit at its feet to prepare for our future.

What we fear varies, but fear itself is not picky. It gladly bolts through any open door to steal ground away from love.

Fear is one of the primary distinctions between viewing faith as a pilgrimage and viewing faith as a performance. Which way do you naturally lean in your view of faith?

A performance is a presentation "in front of an audience,"[5] whereas a pilgrimage is a "journey (usually of a long distance) made to a sacred place as an act of religious devotion; the action or practice of making such a journey."[6] In our context, I am using the term *pilgrimage* not to speak of physical travel, but of spiritual reality. As Paul told the early church, "Our citizenship is in heaven" (Philippians 3:20). In other words, we are not home yet.

Faith viewed as a performance is often motivated by fear and self-protection. Its focus is perfection. Its goal is to avoid even the appearance of failure. If we view faith as a performance, we often see God as a critic, watching our every move with skeptical eyes, red pen in hand, evaluating us by criteria beyond anyone's reach.

As a journey, however, faith viewed as a pilgrimage is motivated by love and glad surrender. Its focus is direction. Its goal is to follow Jesus wherever He leads in the day or the night. If we view faith as a pilgrimage, we will see God as our Companion, Guide, and Destination.

In fact, if we view faith as more of a pilgrimage than a performance, we will see God more than we see ourselves, which is especially helpful when self is what is disillusioning us!

His greatness leads.

Our less-than-greatness follows,

hidden safely (and gratefully) in the bright shadow of His grace.

• • •

Chapter 37

BREATHE DEEPLY

We live in such grace, not because we have earned it (we cannot) and not because we deserve it (we do not), but because of our loving God. He has gone to great extents to gift us with His grace. I wonder how He feels when we reject it.

I wonder how He felt when two of Jesus' first disciples were deciding whether or not to accept it.

Many have noted that the difference between those who ultimately succeed and those who ultimately fail is not that some fail and some do not. Even though the enemy would like us to think that we fail more than others do, in reality, all stumble. The difference in ultimate outcome is determined by *how we respond* to our stumblings.

Applying that wisdom to the darkest night of the disciples' lives, it becomes clear that the difference between Judas and Peter is not that one failed and one did not. Both failed. Additionally, the difference is not that one was disillusioned and one was not. Both Judas and Peter were deeply disillusioned with Jesus and with themselves.

We know that Peter, after denying Jesus, "went outside and wept bitterly" (Luke 22:62). But we sometimes overlook the fact that Judas was also overwhelmed by spiritual pain:

> When Judas, who had betrayed him, saw that Jesus was condemned, he was seized with remorse and returned the thirty silver coins to the chief priests and the elders. "I have sinned," he said, "for I have betrayed innocent blood." "What is that to us?" they replied. "That's your responsibility." So Judas threw the money into the temple and left. Then he went away and hanged himself.
>
> MATTHEW 27:3-5

Both Peter and Judas experienced epic faith fails. Both lost illusions about the strength of their devotion to Jesus. Both gained reality about themselves and their fears. Both knew the night. Yet only one found his way through disillusionment and, greatly humbled, was there to greet Jesus when the sun rose on the third day.

Like Peter, Judas knew he had done wrong. Unlike Peter, Judas confessed Jesus' innocence and his own guilt and even attempted to make restitution by trying to return the payment he had received for betraying Jesus.

The problem is, however, that grace is received, not earned. Grace's pardon cannot be purchased *by* us because it has already been paid *for* us. Our role is to accept it. In order to do so, all illusions of self-redemption must be abandoned.

Whether Judas refused to forgive himself or assumed that God could never forgive him, we do not know. What we do know is that he bailed with finality. When disillusioned with himself, Judas gave up on his faith and his future.

The difference, then, between Judas and Peter is not that one sinned and the other did not, nor that one felt sorrowful and the other felt nothing.

Both sinned. Both felt grieved by their choices. The difference is that when disillusioned, one lost himself in despair and the other found himself in grace.

Grace. Glorious grace.

Grace is what strengthens us to stay committed to our faith walk when disillusioned with ourselves.

Peter showed us the way.

And so, we breathe a sigh of relief when the angel at the tomb says to the women, "Don't be alarmed. You are looking for Jesus the Nazarene, who was crucified. He has risen! He is not here. See the place where they laid him. But go, tell his disciples *and Peter*, 'He is going ahead of you into Galilee. There you will see him, just as he told you'" (Mark 16:6-7, emphasis added).

We cheer as Peter runs to the tomb, goes in, sees "the strips of linen lying there, as well as the burial cloth that had been around Jesus' head" (John 20:6-7) and later, when he jumps out of a boat to get close to Jesus on the shore (see John 21:7).

We hold our breath as Jesus asks Peter three times, "Simon, son of John, do you truly love me more than these?" and Peter, stripped of all pretense by disillusionment with self, finally replies, "Lord, you know all things; you know that I love you" (John 21:15-17).

We nod in agreement when Jesus tells Peter twice, "You must follow me" (John 21:19, 22).

And then we listen with respect as a seasoned Peter, who has followed Jesus through many nights, greets the early church with:

Grace and peace be yours in abundance. Praise be to the God and Father of our Lord Jesus Christ! In his great mercy he has given us new birth into a living hope through the resurrection of Jesus Christ from the dead, and into an inheritance that can never perish, spoil or fade—kept in heaven for you, who through faith are shielded by God's power until the coming of the salvation that is ready to be revealed in the last time.

1 PETER 1:2-5

Peter knew great mercy. He understood what it meant to be "shielded by God's power." He had learned much about abundant grace. And one of his most transformational schools was disillusionment.

Have you ever been disillusioned with yourself? Have you ever lost illusions and gained reality about the frailty of your character, abilities, devotion, or faith?

If so, remember:

Ask God to mentor your mind.

Make sure your signs for spiritual growth are spiritual.

Trade in your line for a spiral.

Critique your definition of victory.

Listen to what God whispers through weakness.

Remember that not all failures are sin.

Give yourself grace to be growing.

And view your faith as a pilgrimage instead of a performance.

For truly it is a pilgrimage—one in which the air is thick with grace.

(Breathe deeply.)

• • •

PART FOUR

Disillusionment with Others

Chapter 38

. . .

(NOT SO) WELL
WITH MY SOUL

We will certainly need to keep deep-breathing grace as we consider the third form of disillusionment: those spaces and seasons in which we say, "Lord, I love You. But Your people are a pain."

Have you ever been disillusioned with Jesus' followers? Have you ever lost illusions and gained reality about life together in the community of faith?

As someone who did not enter that community until adulthood, this form of disillusionment has been the most complicated for me to process. Disillusionment with self and God necessitated navigation through my inner world, which, since I am reflective by nature, was fairly familiar territory. But disillusionment with my newfound Christian family?

Of course, it made sense that imperfect humans would continue to have imperfect relationships on this side of heaven. And it also made sense that each day would be sprinkled with interpersonal losses of illusions and gains of reality like, *Wow. Well, I guess it's best to wait to engage him in conversation until* after *he's had his first cup of coffee.*

But even as a realist, there have been times in my life when disillusionment with God's people took me completely by surprise, like a rug pulled out from underneath me. Flying through the air, I thought, *What on earth just happened?* Landing, I was left with wounds that seemed far more vulnerable to infection than anything I encountered from disillusionment with God or self.

And perhaps I am not alone. Whenever I have the opportunity to ask someone who *used to* consider themselves part of the Church, "What happened? Why did you leave?" most often their responses include some form of disillusionment with God's people.

> *The Church was judgy or hypocritical.*
>
> *The leaders were out-of-touch or too political.*
>
> *No one cared or made room for my gifts.*
>
> *Those I thought were my friends went silent after a rift.*

In short, they did not feel that the people of Jesus acted much like Jesus.

Most of us, since around kindergarten, have understood that the only way to avoid people problems is to avoid people. Life together guarantees drama. But when pain is served to us at God's table, let alone in God's name, we can enter a night that is extremely difficult to negotiate.

Many are familiar with the story behind the classic hymn "It Is Well with My Soul" by Horatio Spafford. But until recently, I was unfamiliar with the story of his disillusionment—not with God or himself, but with God's people.[1]

A vocal opponent of slavery and a successful lawyer, Horatio married Anna Lawson in 1861. Over the next ten years, the couple welcomed four girls to their Chicago home. Since the family invested heavily in real estate, they suffered a devastating financial loss in 1871 when the infamous Great Chicago Fire burned up most of their assets.

Two years later, at the advice of Anna's doctor, Horatio booked passage on a ship to England in the hopes of refreshing his exhausted family (who had been serving others tirelessly in the aftermath of the Chicago fire). Anna and the girls went on ahead, and Horatio planned to follow after attending to some business. While at sea, the steamship sank, and Anna, once safely in England, sent a two-word telegram to Horatio that read, "Saved Alone." All the Spafford children had been lost at sea. On the voyage to bring his Anna back to Chicago, Horatio penned "It Is Well with My Soul" near the spot where his daughters had drowned. The song in itself is stunning, but the backstory places the offering among the greatest anthems of faith in the night.

Grief-stricken, the couple returned home to mourn in the safety of their community of faith. However, instead of finding comfort or even compassion, Horatio

> felt the cold scrutiny of others who dissected his sorrows as if they were specimens to be explained. All Chicago knew the Spaffords had suffered devastating losses in the Great Fire of 1871. The rich, aristocratic young family had been reduced to shabby necessity. Their extravagant plans to visit Europe had been weighed and found wanting. Now, less than two years after the Great Fire, Horatio and Anna had lost all their children. Was this not evidence God was punishing some terrible sin in their lives? Were they not reaping what they had sown?[2]

Though severely disillusioned with God's people, Horatio and Anna chose not to address Job's many "comforters," but instead to mine their pain and make a difference for others by serving the poor.

In 1876, they were blessed with a son, followed by a daughter in 1878 (who would one day carry on their life's work). Tragedy, however, refused to become a stranger. At the age of three or four, their son died from scarlet fever.[3] When they turned to their prayer group for support, one couple actually suggested that the Spaffords give them their only remaining child since they had lost all the others!

Once again, whispers wounded them: "If the Spaffords were true Christians, God would not allow such a thing a second time."[4] Imagine the pain *from around God's table* that they must have known.

As Oswald Chambers once said, "When I suffer and feel I am to blame for it, I can explain it to myself; when I suffer and know I am not to blame, it is a harder matter; but when I suffer and realize that my most intimate relations think I am to blame, that is the limit of suffering."[5]

Surely the Spaffords understood this "limit of suffering." Though they experienced deep interpersonal pain, the couple refused to abandon their God, their faith, or one another.

In fact, it was after this tragedy that Horatio wrote,

> *Long time I dared not say to Thee*
> *O Lord, work Thou Thy will with me,*
> *But now so plain Thy love I see*
> *I shrink no more from sorrow.*
> *So true, true and faithful is He,*
> *Kind is my Savior;*
> *Alike in gladness and in woe,*
> *I thank Him who hath loved me so.*[6]

I shrink no more from sorrow.

After the birth of another daughter in 1881, "the two began making plans to leave the gossips and unfeeling theologians behind, at least for a while. 'We will go to Jerusalem, where Jesus, the Man of Sorrows, lived,' said Horatio."[7] So the family of four left for Jerusalem, where they spent the remainder of their days living . . . *in isolation?* Not at all. In addition to adopting a son, the Spaffords joined with others to plant a community that showed Christ's love to countless souls—Jewish, Christian, and Muslim—by offering generous hospitality, providing food for the poor, and supporting hospitals for the wounded.[8]

As the Spaffords' story illustrates, when disillusioned with God's people, committing to the upward pull of love not only guides us through the night, it keeps our wounds uninfected along the way. Such strength is sourced in faith, not in feelings—the kind of faith Anna Spafford exuded when through the pain she declared, "I will say God is love until I believe it!"[9]

Chapter 39

. . .

SOMETHING OLD
AND SOMETHING NEW

Disillusionment with one another is as old as the Fall. Adam ate the forbidden fruit of his own free will. But when confronted by God about his choice, he blamed his wife before confessing to his own complicity: "The woman you put here with me—she gave me some fruit from the tree, and I ate it" (Genesis 3:12). Though God and Eve knew the whole story, I do wonder how Eve felt when her husband threw her under the proverbial bus instead of taking responsibility for his part in the transgression.

From that point forward in Scripture, more chapters than not recount or evidence some level of interpersonal pain, from tension in the first marriage in Genesis 3 to the mysterious end-times drama described in the book of Revelation. For example,

Cain, in a rage, kills Abel.

Noah, with a hangover, curses his son Ham.

Abraham lies and calls his wife, Sarah, his sister.

Sarah uses Hagar and then has her sent into the desert to die.

Isaac, like his father, passes his wife off as his sister to save his own skin.

Jacob deceives Isaac to receive his elder brother's blessing.

Joseph is sold into slavery by his siblings, only later to rise in political power and show mercy to his guilt-laden (and more than a little nervous) brothers.

And that just brings us to the end of the first book of the Bible!

Though Old Testament examples abound (David's life alone could easily fill a multi-season melodrama), we will return to our standing example in Psalm 42. In addition to being disillusioned with God and himself, this son of Korah was also disillusioned with the people around him:

My tears have been my food day and night, while people say to me all day long, "Where is your God?"
PSALM 42:3

My bones suffer mortal agony as my foes taunt me, saying to me all day long, "Where is your God?"
PSALM 42:10

King David loved God and was leading his nation in devotion to God. As David's musician and psalmist, this son of Korah would have been surrounded by others who, like himself, were in or near King David's inner circle. However, God's people can be clumsy, and sometimes even cruel, in handling one another's pain. When this psalmist desperately needed encouragement, those near him—friends and foes alike in David's court—only added to his agony.

The New Testament also is replete with interpersonal conflicts, misunderstandings, and betrayals *within* the community of faith. I emphasize *within* because that is our focus. As we consider biblical examples and then turn our attention to eleven tools that will help us to navigate this form of spiritual night, our context is disillusionment with others who share our belief in and devotion to Jesus.

In other words, this is not about random road rage, religious freedom, problems with the pagans next door, or the resident wolf in sheep's clothing. This is about interpersonal disillusionment among those who are trying to follow Jesus.

This is when . . .

> Jesus asked the disciples, "'What were you arguing about on the road?' But they kept quiet because on the way they had argued about who was the greatest" (Mark 9:33-34).

> Peter, speaking of John, asked Jesus, "Lord, what about him?" (John 21:21).

> Ananias and Sapphira lied to the apostles (Acts 5:1-11).

> Grecian Jews in the early church "complained against the Hebraic Jews because their widows were being overlooked in the daily distribution of food" (Acts 6:1).

> A gloriously saved Paul went to Jerusalem and "tried to join the disciples, but they were all afraid of him, not believing that he really was a disciple" (Acts 9:26).

> Paul said to Barnabas, "'Let us go back and visit the brothers in all the towns where we preached the word of the Lord and see how they are doing.' Barnabas wanted to take John, also called Mark, with them, but Paul did not think it wise to take him, because he had deserted them in Pamphylia and had not continued with them in the work. They had such a sharp disagreement that they parted company" (Acts 15:36-39).

> Peter came to Antioch and Paul "opposed him to his face, because he was clearly in the wrong. Before certain men came from James, he used to eat with the Gentiles. But when they arrived, he began to draw back and separate himself from the Gentiles because he was afraid of those who belonged to the circumcision group. The other Jews joined him in his hypocrisy, so

that by their hypocrisy even Barnabas was led astray" (Galatians 2:11-13).

Paul confessed to his spiritual son, Timothy, "At my first defense, no one came to my support, but everyone deserted me. May it not be held against them" (2 Timothy 4:16).

Ambition, comparison, mistrust, hypocrisy, deception, favoritism, division, abandonment—sometimes we romanticize the early church, but they were no strangers to this type of spiritual pain.

Just like them, we too can experience disillusionment within the community of faith when . . .

A friend elevates themselves by putting you down.

A spiritual leader has a moral failure.

You pay the price for a friend's jealousy.

Someone you know slanders someone you love.

You feel doubted by the very people who once championed you.

The soul who led you to Jesus loses their faith in God.

The people you came to serve are not excited about your service.

You were not invited to this committee or that party.

Someone drops the ball and now you look irresponsible.

Others suddenly start avoiding you, and you do not know why.

You confide in someone who proceeds to betray your confidence.

A frenemy is given an opportunity you thought you had earned.

Your name is stained by someone else's sin.

Acquaintances know little and assume much.

You feel undervalued or overlooked by those who know you best.

Others blatantly refuse to see or tell the truth.

Does any of this feel familiar?

When we experience disillusionment with God, the good news is that He is perfect, so the challenge is one-sided (ours). However, when we experience disillusionment with each other, the situation is far more complex. In this type of night, there are (at least) two imperfect humans with illusions, both of whom have free wills and neither of whom have any guarantee that the other will not bail.

Chapter 40

...

SUNDAY
SCHOOLED

We have been designed, from the very beginning, to be in community. All of us naturally long for relationship with one another and ultimately, with God. What was true at Creation when God was gifting Adam with Eve and said, "It is not good for the man to be alone" (Genesis 2:18) is still true today. In the words of Solomon in Ecclesiastes 4:9-10, "Two are better than one, because they have a good return for their work: If one falls down, his friend can help him up. But pity the man who falls and has no one to help him up!"

Truly, two are better than one.

And . . . two are more complicated than one.

Jesus understood this well. His hand-chosen leadership team was comprised of men with significant differences politically, socially, and perhaps even theologically. From Simon the Zealot to Matthew the tax collector, from James and John, Sons of Thunder, to Peter the rock, Jesus collected quite a combustible crew.

Then, at the Last Supper, on the threshold of the most disillusioning days that the disciples would ever experience, Jesus announced, "A new command I give you: Love one another. As I have loved you, so you must love one another. By this all men will know that you are my disciples, if you love one another" (John 13:34-35).

Early in His public ministry, Jesus told the crowds to "love your enemies" (Matthew 5:44). Now, toward the end of His public ministry, Jesus commanded His closest followers to "love one another." Something of eternal weight—i.e., "all men will know"—rested (and still rests) on what is sometimes referred to as the eleventh commandment.

Seated around the table that evening were disciples on the verge of deep disillusionment with Jesus, themselves, and each other. Judas would betray them. Jesus would allow Himself to be taken from them. Satan would sift them. Panic would grip them. Fear would expose them. The crucifixion would stun them. And grief would overcome them.

How on earth could they possibly navigate such spiritual pain?

Together.

Through love.

Of all the things Jesus could have said at the Last Supper to guide them, He left them with one clear command: love each other, all the way through the night.

In the 1960s, Peter Raymond Scholtes wrote a song based on this command that has since been covered by many artists. The first two verses of the original lyrics read as follows:

> *We are one in the Spirit, we are one in the Lord.*
> *We are one in the Spirit, we are one in the Lord.*
> *And we pray that all unity may one day be restored.*
> *And they'll know we are Christians by our love, by our love.*
> *Yes, they'll know we are Christians by our love.*
> *We will walk with each other, we will walk hand in hand.*

We will walk with each other, we will walk hand in hand,
And together we'll spread the news that God is in our land.
And they'll know we are Christians by our love, by our love.
Yes, they'll know we are Christians by our love.[1]

Amen.

But *how?*

In part, by actively resisting the way of hate. When we consider the audience of John 13, Jesus' "love one another" clearly did not mean that His followers would always agree about everything. Love is the fruit, not of sameness but of commitment. Even when we do not see eye to eye, we can still commit to Jesus' upward call of love for each other. Perhaps to Simon the Zealot and Matthew the tax collector, Jesus was saying, "Keep loving, even if you never start liking." Perhaps to Paul and Barnabas, He was saying, "Keep loving, even when you choose to part ways."

As we lose illusions and gain reality about one another, love is Jesus' call to us. It is pure and purifying, challenging and death-defying. It can lift us beyond the heights of our humanity even when we are in the depths of despair.

And, grievously, this sacred call of Jesus has also been twisted out of context and misquoted to rationalize injustice, enable abusers, and silence the oppressed. I am painfully aware that you, brave reader, may carry deep wounds from treatment you were told to tolerate in the name of love. Jesus' eleventh commandment has sometimes been weaponized within the Church to bully victims into submission. Slaveholders, spouse beaters, and sickly leaders alike have sought to spiritualize passivity in those they mistreat in the name of love that "bears all things" (1 Corinthians 13:7, ESV).

This was not the message of John 13, and it is not the message of this book. As we now turn our attention toward tools to help us navigate disillusionment within the family of God, let us remember their intended context: not wolves in sheep's clothing, but fellow imperfect, in-process, and occasionally wounded sheep, whose hearts are set on following Jesus all the way Home.

Deciding *which* tools to offer you here has been quite a challenge. I have sorted and rearranged, omitted and organized the possibilities again and again. In the end, what follows is a fusion of *skills* to help you deescalate (and perhaps even prevent) painful drama in the family of faith and *principles* to help you choose the way of love (toward God, others, and yourself) when interpersonal pain is unavoidable.

WHEN DISILLUSIONED WITH GOD'S PEOPLE, BE SLOW TO ASSUME THAT SIN IS THE SOURCE.

Yes, we are sinners. And yes, our sin is a significant source of interpersonal disillusionment. We are all painfully aware of this reality.

But *life* also does a magnificent job manufacturing drama "all by its lonesome" (as my Mississippi-born dad used to say). In fact, plain old life may be the most active, yet least recognized, source of disillusionment around God's table.

We are different people from different places with different pasts, pains, and personalities. Add to that mix different cultures and generations, and it is a miracle that we ever understand each other at all. Life itself—its diversity, complexity, and constant change—accounts for a great deal of our misunderstandings.

Even *before* we add in sin.

My first missionary assignments were in Singapore, Hong Kong, and Indonesia. From the people to the food, life looked different, so it was natural for me to anticipate difference. Consequently, I experienced far less culture shock in Asia than I did during my next assignment in Australia, where life down under did not, on the surface, seem that dissimilar from life back in the States.

Some of my dearest friends on the planet today are Australian, so clearly, we all survived my many missteps. But at the start of my time there, I felt so out of place and out of step with the culture that I joined an expat Asian church to gain a sense of grounding.

One day during Sunday school, the teacher shared a principle that helped me despiritualize a lot of the interpersonal disillusionment I was facing. Dividing the room in two on opposite sides of a table, he had each group face each other while he drew a large number in chalk on the table in between.

Turning to the first group, he asked, "What number is this?"

In unison we responded, "A six."

Turning to the other group, he asked again, "What number is this?"

In unison they replied, "A nine."

"Are either of you *wrong*?" he pressed.

Shaking our heads, we all lifted our eyes from the number on the table to the souls on the other side of the table and answered, "No."

Point made.

Lesson learned.

(Or, at least, lesson heard).

When you grow up in the same house (physically or spiritually) but on different sides of the table, disagreements are not always stirred up by

Satan or sourced in personal sin. Yes, the enemy "prowls around like a roaring lion looking for someone to devour" (1 Peter 5:8). And without question, our sin pains Christ and His church.

But more often than we may imagine, our interpersonal disillusionment is sourced in plain old *life*—life together as the family of God.

Chapter 41

. . .

LESS THAN
BLESSED

The repercussions of being an only child honestly were not on my radar until I became a parent and suddenly realized that I had no built-in uncles and aunties to contribute to the equation. Thankfully, Barry added a loving sister, and God generously filled in the circle with extraordinary souls who have surrounded our three since their births.

One auntie, who will remain unnamed (Jennifer Day), "gifted" our firstborn *preschooler* with a monstrous—excuse me, I mean marvelous—electronic drum set complete with twangy tunes, preset drum patterns, and a volume control that was clearly designed to provide listening pleasure for all within a block radius.

This auntie, who will not be named (Jennifer Day), brought her gift joyfully into our house. However, our gifts are not always others' blessings. Which seems a fitting lead-in to our next tool.

WHEN DISILLUSIONED WITH GOD'S PEOPLE,
HUMBLY ACKNOWLEDGE THAT YOUR STRENGTHS
MIGHT HAVE SHADOWS.

We tend to think more about shadows of sin than shadows of strengths. For example, if someone has a jealous nature, all near them have to live and work in the shadow of that jealousy. This type of complication to life together is somewhat obvious.

Strength shadows, however, are a less intuitive source of disillusionment because it rarely occurs to us that our giftings could supply anything other than blessing to a relationship.

This next exercise is especially entertaining in a group. (I trust that it will still be of benefit to you as a reader.) To help us process disillusionment from a slightly different angle, I would like to invite you to do two things. First, consider what shadows might accompany the following types of strengths:

Detailed money managers

Creative artists

Skilled communicators

Gifted listeners

Visionary leaders

Loyal administrators

Second, now that you have warmed up your strength-shadow detectors, I encourage you to pause further reading to answer the following three questions:

1. What are some of your strengths? (Phone a friend if you get stuck.)
2. What are some of the shadows that occasionally accompany your strengths? (Phone a friend if you dare.)
3. What are the names of the souls who have to live or work in the shadow of your strengths? (Pray for them . . . regularly.)

While you are at it, you can add my husband to your prayers. I am an analytical troubleshooter who married a servant-hearted visionary. Though people may prize my troubleshooting giftings when in need of a mentor, consultant, or teacher, that same gift may drive them, well, *nuts* if all they really want to do is decide, for example, where to put the coffeepot. Such a decision is slowed down, but rarely aided, by my offer of a dozen different scenarios with correlating consequences.

When I married Barry, no one told me that true visionaries dream as a form of relaxation. So, when Barry released a dozen ideas a day into the atmosphere as though he were hosting a hot-air balloon festival, I would "help" him by pulling out my troubleshooting strength and blasting those balloons out of the sky with my realism. A nicer person by nature than me, Barry at first felt surprised, then confused, and ultimately shut down. He was living in the shadow of my strengths.

Thankfully, well before our shared disillusionment could become disastrous, God intervened and showed me that my strength-shadows were causing Barry to question how God had made him. "Let the boy dream, Alicia!" God said. "He's not dreaming *to do*; he's dreaming *to be*. He's dreaming *with Me*."

Barry forgave me, but frankly, it took a while to rebuild what I had torn down. The lesson stuck with me and has eased my way through disillusionment with God's people too many times to count.

Another way to consider this concept of strength shadows and its contribution to disillusionment is with a contrast I crafted a few decades ago. In advance, I confess: what follows is not scientific. It has no citations. I have not consulted a neuropsychologist or even a good book on interpersonal conflict. Though simplistic, the contrast has consistently proven helpful to others, so I am going to risk offering it here to you.

It seems to me that all of us are motivated by the need *to produce* (to make things of value), *to relate* (to have meaningful relationships), and *to think* (to process life and its complexities). Envision these three motivations as a rotating (not fixed) cluster. The flexibility is important because different motivations can take the lead in different circumstances and seasons. For example, a different motivation may take the lead when you are in charge of a project than when you are supporting someone else who is in charge of a project. Or that cluster may shift as you transition with a parent from the role of dependent to the role of caregiver.

Even so, we all can probably identify one motivation that tends to take the lead within us more often. For example, whereas my husband is more of a relater/thinker, I am more of a thinker/relater. (And yes, we hire someone to do our taxes.)

In general, producers tend to:

> start the day with a to-do list
>
> value the visible and the measurable
>
> emphasize efficiency and results
>
> be stressed by discussion that does not end in decision
>
> go to the office on their day off
>
> feel guilty or bored taking a vacation

Relaters tend to:

> start the day by checking in (via texts or socials) with their clos-est hundred friends
>
> prize relationships above all else
>
> emphasize community and faithfulness
>
> feel stressed when others put tasks before people

visit with coworkers (a lot) to make sure they know they are seen and important

feel working with people they love IS a vacation

Thinkers tend to:

start the day with, well, themselves

view thinking as a form of relaxation

emphasize process and integrity

feel stressed by phrases like "Let's just wing it!"

press for constant evaluation of motives and methods

wish that everyone else would go on vacation so they could think in peace

Imagine with me all the potential combinations that exist within your family, cohort of coworkers, office team, staff members, or friendship groups. The table below attempts to capture how each primary motivation might view the others.

	Look at producers and say . . .	Look at relaters and say . . .	Look at thinkers and say . . .
Producers	Jesus was a change-agent. We producers are the ones who really make things happen.	If you really care as much as you say you do, stop talking and start helping!	Wake me up when you're ready to DO something.
Relaters	The only thing we can really take with us in life are relationships. You are more important than anything you can produce.	Jesus was a relater. We relaters prioritize people over tasks.	Chill, my friend. You are suffering from severe brain strain. Come up for air and have some fun.
Thinkers	I know you find value in activity. But are you really in touch with the *why* behind the *what* that you do?	One question: Don't you ever need to be *alone*?	Jesus was the ultimate thinker and strategist. We thinkers wrestle with the real issues of life.

Built-in drama!

So perhaps we can laugh a bit more and blame sin a bit less for the challenges we face as a community. Plain old *life* and *strength shadows* confirm the innate complexity of life together *before* anything else even enters the room.

Chapter 42

. . .

HOW WE HEAR

"And above all, please interpret his words and his actions through his heart."

This request is one I have made repeatedly over the years as an advocate for my eldest son. Whenever he enters a new environment—in school, at church, on mission trips, at work—we ask for the opportunity to share about high-functioning autism in general and Jonathan in particular.

Jonathan's heart is almost always in the right place. He is among the most tender, loyal, grateful, and honest souls that I have ever known. Graced with a brilliant mind and a compassionate heart, Jonathan loves being with others. But when those others are quick to make assumptions and slow to ask clarifying questions, the interpersonal pain of being misunderstood or falsely accused overwhelms Jonathan to the point of shutdown. When people have heard his heart poorly, my son has been wounded severely. In fact, when I asked him for permission to share this story, Jonathan said, "Oh, yes! Please do. Thank you, Mom!"

Honestly, learning to hear others' hearts more loudly than their words is a skill that would help us all.

WHEN DISILLUSIONED WITH GOD'S PEOPLE, LEARN TO LISTEN GENEROUSLY.

Generous listening is becoming a lost art. Perhaps because listening, in general, has become a lost skill. As a culture, we now collect information in clips and bits that are rarely, if ever, capable of capturing the complexities of a human heart.

Whether we are hearing, hard of hearing, or deaf, whether we communicate through spoken words, print, or sign language, our ability to truly hear one another seems to have decreased even though our ability to instantly access one another has significantly increased.

Sacrificing quality for quickness, we are shouting louder, but fewer of us seem to feel *heard*.

Hearing others is not equally easy for all. From ADHD to OCD, from trauma to tinnitus, some have more internal noise to navigate than others. Thankfully, listening from the heart is a skill, and whatever our starting point, as a skill it can be developed.

We can begin by not treating parts as though they were wholes. What we hear, read, or see is just a piece, just a percentage of what others are saying, thinking, and feeling. It is baffling today how we expect one another to account for all truth in one tweet, or post, or even speech. Generous listening knows there is always more to the story and hears what is offered for what it really is: one part of a bigger picture.

Generous listening also hears for others' sake as much as for our own. Sometimes we are a bit mercenary in our listening, mining conversations for only what benefits us. We listen, but to gather information to strengthen our side. We listen, but then selectively sort through all the words to piece together evidence of our woes. We listen to take, to use, and to triumph instead of listening *as a gift* to others and to ourselves.

Another aspect of generous listening is the choice to pause before personalizing others' words. Since my kids were small, they have heard me say repeatedly, "Others' behaviors and words tell you more about them than about yourselves."

"Yes, Mama," they often reply, "but it still hurts."

"Absolutely," I empathize, "and what did you learn about *them?*"

Even with more than a few decades' practice, this still is not completely natural for me. I cannot count the number of times that I have practiced controlled breathing while listening to someone and simultaneously telling myself, *This is their anxiety (or disappointment or rejection, etc.) speaking. This is not really about me at all.* Of course, humility invites us to learn about ourselves from others' lenses, but personalizing everything does not help anyone be truly heard.

And though it may be obvious, there is one more aspect I want to emphasize: generous listening lets others *speak.* Changing subjects, cutting people off, and tuning people out is a surefire way to stoke unnecessary drama. Perhaps this is one of the reasons we sometimes prefer texting to talking and posting online to processing face-to-face: we can express ourselves without interaction or interruption and let others read and respond (or not).

Developing the skill to hear others' hearts more loudly than their words is not easy. It is a lifelong effort requiring self-control, focus, and patience. But imagine the unnecessary disillusionment we would avoid—and imagine the actual disillusionment we would ease—if we could simply slow down and truly try to hear one another. Surely all our relationships would benefit from any effort we exert to grow as generous listeners.

Chapter 43

HOLDING
THE GLASS

One of the reasons that so many individuals with high-functioning autism carry such deep interpersonal scars is related to the expectations of those who interact with them. Without question, social challenges are faced by everyone who has special needs. However, early on, I realized that because Jonathan does not wear his special needs on the outside, people expect him to think and interact "typically." Consequently, if he, for example, misses a nonverbal cue or has difficulty following multistep directions, others' confusion or disappointment is amplified.

The illustration that comes to mind is that of a glass falling onto the floor. If the distance between the glass and floor is minimal, the glass will probably remain intact. However, if the distance between the glass and floor is substantial, the glass will surely shatter.

Taking the time to identify how high above reality we are holding the glasses of our interpersonal expectations is a wise use of energy, especially in the night.

WHEN DISILLUSIONED WITH GOD'S PEOPLE,
ARTICULATE YOUR EXPECTATIONS.

The presence of expectations is a prerequisite for the loss of illusions. Even when we sincerely believe we have no expectations, this is rarely true. What *is* true is that there are different kinds of expectations, some of which are more obvious than others.

Some expectations are *unknown* (which is not a synonym for *nonexistent*). These assumptions are so deep within us that we do not even know they exist until life calls them into question, and stunned, we think, *What? But I was sure that everyone . . .*

The discovery of some can be humorous, like when a friend tells us they think chocolate tastes like dirt and we are speechless. Why? Because an unknown expectation—i.e., that all reasonable souls possess an innate appreciation of all things cocoa bean—was just revealed and refuted.

The discovery of other unknown expectations, however, is not funny at all. Throughout my college years, I was graced with mentors both at home and at school. Meeting with a mentor once a week was just discipleship-as-usual to me. After graduating and moving overseas, I waited at least a week to get past jet lag before going into a leader's office and asking him who my mentor would be. Puzzled, he asked, "Your mentor?"

Hmm, I thought, *Maybe this culture uses a different word.* So I offered, "Oh, I'm sorry, I mean my discipler. Um, spiritual coach?"

He replied, "Are you troubled?"

"Well, not really," I said. "You know like how Jesus had the twelve disciples? Or how Paul told Timothy, 'The things you have heard me say in the presence of many witnesses entrust to reliable men who will also be qualified to teach others'?" (2 Timothy 2:2, NIV).

"Ah," he said as he picked up the phone to make an appointment for me *with a therapist.*

I was dumbfounded because I had stumbled upon an unknown expectation. I thought the entire global Church was one big, happy, mentoring family. I had no clue that my experience was more the exception than the rule.

Other expectations are known, but *unstated*, most often because we feel they are too obvious to warrant repeating. Like when you take a job with a friend and expect that, working side by side, you will become even better friends. Then when you learn that Joe-as-just-your-buddy was a lot nicer than Joe-as-your-new-boss, the distance is disillusioning. Or when you have an unstated expectation, like *Real friends celebrate one another's birthday.* Then, when a friend sends you a text the day after your birthday instead of throwing you a party on your big day, you feel disappointed. Such unstated expectations, though jolting, are still easier to recover from than a third type of expectation.

Interpersonally, the most dangerous expectations are those that are *unshared.* Though known and stated, these expectations are incompatible and can lead to painful impasses if both sides cannot find a creative work-around. Like when you thought someone joined the team to support your dream, but they think your dream is a waste of time. This is not just a matter of saying the same thing with different words. Unshared expectations come from differently sourced (and not always complementary) values.

Though some expectations can only take us by surprise, spending time identifying the rest is a wise relational investment. So, when you enter a new environment or a different season, sit down with Jesus and ask for His help in articulating your expectations as specifically as you can. Write them down. Process them in prayer. Ask God for life-giving edits as needed. Identified and evaluated, our expectations can be held a little closer to the ground of reality, which can lead to less shattering for all involved.

Chapter 44

· · ·

TABLE
STRETCHES

Disillusionment in the community of faith is not evidence of failed relationships. It is evidence of *existing* relationships. Though a poor comparison, this is an immediate one to me. Outside my writing room window, one of our dogs is barking rhythmically, as though he is keeping time with some distant (but not distant enough) song.

I wish I did not notice, but I do. I wish it did not bother me, but it does. The dog, however, has not failed. He is just being a doggy. His barks are evidence of his existence. (Ours are, too.) My dog cannot change how he barks, so it is left to me to change *how I respond*. All of which leads to our next encouragement.

WHEN DISILLUSIONED WITH GOD'S PEOPLE,
CULTIVATE MENTAL FLEXIBILITY.

One summer, when Keona was little, I signed us up for a private ballet class. It was just the two of us plus an incredible instructor named Kim. By way of full disclosure, I let Kim know from the start that I was not very flexible and never had been. My perspective on flexibility was that its bandwidth was probably set at birth, and mine was genetically narrow. Kim smiled and explained that if you can move, you can always become more flexible because flexibility is not fixed. Evidently, expanding our flexibility does the body a world of good at any age.

Mental flexibility[1] is not dissimilar. The field of neuroscience is exploding with good news about the brain's plasticity and our ability to keep learning and creating new pathways well past what once was considered the golden learning years of youth. Whether or not we naturally feel mentally flexible, our brains are wired for growth.

And growing will strengthen the body of Christ.

A good starting place is agreeing to disagree. Not in the name of relativism nor in the name of apathy, but rather in the name of love. As I listen to pain in the community of faith, rarely (if ever) have I heard anyone say that their interpersonal pain was sourced in theological disagreements about Christ's deity or the nature of salvation, but rather in how they were *treated*.

In light of that reality, when it comes to issues that are not a matter of heaven and hell, could we give ourselves permission to see things differently? Does every question have one and only one reasonable answer? Must someone always have to win? Might there be value in ties or even occasional losses?

Mental flexibility would enable us to disagree and then still go enjoy dinner together. Instead, our threshold for disagreement is so low that at the first sign of not being on the same page, we block, cancel, and bail on one another for issues that, even if real, may not be eternal.

Mental flexibility protects us from relational extremism (i.e., "One strike and you're out.") and overreactions (i.e., "If you disagree with my idea, you're really disagreeing with my existence."). It empowers us to redefine relational victory in terms of the shared pursuit of truth and respect, as opposed to cold, countable wins and losses.

This, in turn, positively affects our ability to process pushback and criticism. We say we want feedback, but in practice, perhaps what we really want are thumbs-up and hearts. Our lack of mental flexibility is revoking our freedom to simply be honest.

Surely all generations would assert that they value both honesty and unity. But the differences in how we define and order those terms causes more than a little disillusionment in the Church. Some define *honesty* as self-expression and, as such, believe that self-expression should be sacrificed for the sake of unity. Others feel it is impossible to really have unity without the freedom to be entirely honest. Still others are fine with honesty as long as it is complimentary toward them and never labeled *truth*.

Therefore, within the family of God, some are offended because they view being questioned as a sign of disrespect, others feel obligated to be brutally truthful in their pursuit of unity, and still others interpret the least sign of criticism as rejection. And while we expend our energy overreacting to one another, the truly great commission God has entrusted to us (see Matthew 28:18-20) goes unattended.

Sad for us?

Yes.

But it is especially unfortunate for those we are supposed to be serving.

Sometimes, when I am disillusioned with one of God's kids, *picturing us both at God's table* helps me cultivate mental flexibility. Our memories may not be in agreement about a conflict. Our core values may be out of alignment. Our priorities may compete. But we are equally at the table only through the merciful invitation of our Host, whom we both call God and Savior.

Could I, should I, dare I make a case to Father God as to why this other soul should not be at His table in heaven?

If not, then perhaps I should mentally stretch toward them a bit more here on earth.

Chapter 45

• • •

TO HAVE,
OR NOT TO HAVE,
A COW

The story has stayed with me for years. Dear friends[1] were out of town, and their incredibly responsible high school sons were taking care of the house and ranch. Somehow, one of their cows fell into a neighbor's pool. Waking up at the neighbor's knocking, the eldest went to check out the situation and then hurried back to get his brother's help. Their interaction went something like this:

Eldest (wide awake): Hey, get up! I need your help.

Youngest (mostly asleep): Why? What's up?

Eldest: One of the cows fell into the neighbor's pool. It's really cold, and we need to get it out quick. I can't do it alone.

Youngest (pausing to think): *Whose* cow is it?

Eldest: What?

Youngest: Whose cow is it?

Eldest: Well, it's *my* cow.

Youngest (rolling back over onto his pillow): Not my cow. Not my problem.

WHEN DISILLUSIONED WITH GOD'S PEOPLE,
KNOW WHEN IT IS NOT YOUR COW.

The rest of the story is that the youngest did get up to help his elder brother, and the cow survived (I think). But the younger brother's response is close to a textbook example of *differentiation*.

The first time I came across this term was in my doctoral studies through the writings of psychologist Edwin H. Friedman. Friedman defines differentiation as

> the capacity of a family member to define his or her own life's goals and values apart from surrounding togetherness pressures, to say "I" when others are demanding "you" and "we." It includes the capacity to maintain a (relatively) nonanxious presence in the midst of anxious systems, to take maximum responsibility for one's own destiny and emotional being. It can be measured somewhat by the breadth of one's repertoire of responses when confronted with crisis. The concept should not be confused with autonomy or narcissism, however. Differentiation means the capacity to be an "I" while remaining connected.[2]

(And all the therapists, psychologists, counselors, and mentors reading this book just said, "Yes. Yes, and amen!")

Differentiation is the ability to know what is and what is not your cow. It does not mean that we disconnect or never help others, but rather, that our choice to help does not emanate from confusion about what is and is not our responsibility.

Though some souls rarely assume responsibility for anything (i.e., nothing is ever their fault or issue), this principle is more for those of us who tend to assume responsibility for everything (i.e., we are taking care of everyone's cows).

In the context of disillusionment with others, differentiation makes us less vulnerable to being manipulated by the power of others' emotions. Knowing where we end and others begin helps us find enough ground to stand upon and make decisions based on accuracy instead of felt urgency.

Many years before Friedman's book gifted me with the term, a wise, older friend enlightened me with the concept. I was feeling troubled in a newer friendship with someone whom she had known for a long, long time. "She's a wonderful person," I began, "but I cannot seem to make a connection. I feel like she's always displeased with me."

My perceptions were only partly accurate. Yes, she had not hidden her view that my work did not qualify as a real job. And I knew (but did not disclose) that her job, though extremely valuable, would bore me to tears. But what I had not accounted for—and would not see for years to come—was the extreme differences in our families of origin. She had been raised that *to affirm* was *to spoil*. I had been raised that *to affirm* was *to empower*.

Nonetheless, the relationship was valuable to me, and I had hit a wall in knowing how to build a bridge. Our mutual friend listened to me, nodded knowingly, and then said, "Alicia, people come with their stuff, and they will leave with their stuff. You didn't give it to them, and you can't take it away from them."

With a fabulous fusion of mercy and wisdom, she was encouraging me to realize that there were other issues at play beyond my current view. Since I did not cause them, I could not dissolve them. (In short, not my cow.)

It is counterintuitive how freeing it is to finally accept that some things (like other people's opinions and emotions) are outside of our control. Doing so opens the way for us to offer others the "nonanxious presence" mentioned by Friedman. I cannot overemphasize how much working on this skill has helped me in processing disillusionment as a daughter and parent, a friend and spouse, an employee and employer. Attempting to correct emotion by adding more emotion is rarely effective. Yet how often do we respond to others' anxiety by becoming anxious? How often do we react to others' stress by becoming stressed? It is like adding fuel to a fire and wondering why it does not go out.

Jesus is the ultimate example of this ability to remain calm in the midst of others' storms. From sleeping in the boat during a tempest (see Matthew 8:23-27) to being silent before Herod (see Luke 23:8-15), Jesus could not be controlled by others' fears or fancies. And He is the One who says to us,

> Come to me, all you who are weary and burdened, and I will give you rest. Take my yoke upon you and learn from me, for I am gentle and humble in heart, and you will find rest for your souls. For my yoke is easy and *my burden is light*.
> MATTHEW 11:28-30, EMPHASIS ADDED

(Other people's cows are not.)

Chapter 46

· · ·

A MUSCULAR
MERCY

Her name was Rebekka, and she is now in her Savior's embrace.

For twenty years I was graced to count her among my mentors. She prayed for me daily, and every year, we enjoyed one glorious hour face-to-face during my annual prayer retreats at Canaan in the Desert,[1] where she lived and served. Sitting in a quiet room, Rebekka listened to whatever happened to be the heaviest weight on my heart. Pausing, she would then offer prayerful thoughts wrapped in her soft German accent. Each time, I journaled our talks and would feast on the wisdom God gave to me through her for months.

Or, in this instance, for the rest of my life.

What was on my heart that year was not heavy; it was devastating. I was disillusioned with God's people. The pain had leveled me emotionally. It was the longest and thickest night I had ever known.

Able to discern some of the sources, a part of me wanted to confront the issues, to expose the errors, to set the record straight. After all, is it not the truth that sets us free? But I knew there was too much hurt in my heart for it to be wise to speak . . . yet.

"Not now, but one day soon," I said, expressing my frustration to Rebekka.

Characteristically, she thought awhile and then said, "My dear Alicia, let me tell you a story. There once was a man who was weary of discovering his sins day after day and year after year. So, he prayed and asked God to show him all his sins at once. God replied, 'Oh, My son, My son, if I were to show you everything that I see, you would surely die.'"

We sat in silence while the story sank in, and then she added, "Alicia, God's mercy is stronger than His truth."

Feel free to be startled by her statement. (It certainly offended me.)

What? I thought. *Nothing is stronger than God's truth!* However, in the context of relationships, Rebekka was right: because of God's mercy, He does not reveal *all that is true* about us *all at once.* His mercy restrains His truth, rationing out revelation since its fullness would crush us.

The lesson was clear without her saying another word. God, in His love, does not instantly tell us everything that is true about us. He sees more than He says. Mercy guides both His speech and His silence. And I needed to follow His example.

WHEN DISILLUSIONED WITH GOD'S PEOPLE, SPEAK TO HEAL, NOT TO HARM.

I had assumed that insight always implied invitation—that if I saw something, it was just a matter of time before I was supposed to say something. But speaking is not always the commission of seeing. Sometimes we are entrusted with insight so that we can pray and show mercy, not so that we can confront and correct.

Of course, God's speech *can* still hurt. In the Gospels, surely Jesus' rebukes stung. But even when aimed at hypocrites—for whom Jesus reserved His harshest speech[2]—the sting of His words was surgical, whether or not those who heard His words wanted to be healed.

When disillusioned with God's people, and given God's permission to speak, how can our words heal instead of harm? Several principles can guide us.

First, before speaking, ask yourself why you are really speaking. For good? For God? To vent? To purge? To avenge? To save face? Being honest before God with what is motivating your desire to speak will help you pause long enough to get in step with His desires.

Second, if given God's green light to speak, minimize drama by maximizing respect. Speak *to them* instead of *to others about them*. Use more "I" words than "you" words. For example, "This is how *I* felt when . . ." instead of "This is how *you* made me feel when . . ." As they respond, listen to learn, not to gather ammunition. God is the Creator of everyone you meet. In difficult conversations, respecting others as God's workmanship may or may not soften their hearts, but it will position you to learn all you can in the situation.

Third, if you need to correct, do not clothe it in humor. Used as a hint, humor can be a type of avoidance or manipulation. This lesson came home to me through the honesty of an eighteen-year-old college student whom I will call Maria. Maria had begun dating a leader in our ministry, and the two of them were at our house watching a movie together. The TV was in the loft, and, as I was cleaning the dishes down in the kitchen after dinner, my concern about their closeness on the couch kept increasing. Heading up to the loft with my husband, I quipped with a laugh, "All right everyone, the married couple is here. We have dibs on the couch!" It was barely humorous and even less honest, but the two moved obligingly onto some chairs. *Mission accomplished*, I thought, oblivious to what was awaiting me after the movie's end.

"Alicia," Maria began. "Can I talk with you?"

"Sure," I said with forced calm.

She continued, "Were you uncomfortable with how close I was sitting to my boyfriend on the couch?"

"Um, well—" My mind raced. "Now that you mention it, I suppose I was, a little."

"Is that why you made that joke about the couch?" she asked.

"Hmm. I suppose they were related," I admitted sheepishly.

Maria paused and then schooled me. "Alicia, I expect you to be a woman of God. If you have something to say to me, *just say it.*"

Ouch. But a good ouch. She was right. Humor as a hint more often damages trust than actually instructs.

And fourth, to help words heal instead of harm, limit your circle of advisers and sympathizers. In other words, be careful whom you invite into your offense. This is not remotely an endorsement of isolation, but rather an encouragement to seek counsel from emotionally mature souls.

When disillusioned with God's people, you need a few wise, safe sounding boards, not a slew of subjective, hyper-protective friends. Avoid potential candidates who post publicly everything they think privately, who value your acceptance more than they value the truth, or who have a history of proving their love for you by removing their love from others.

Instead, search for generous listeners who can hear without getting huffy, empathize without being paralyzed, and still be objective enough to help you consider how things might look from the other side.

Though these parameters might narrow the field of potential advisers significantly, truly wise counsel can reduce the harm our words can cause substantially.

Chapter 47

WHAT WAS, WAS

When disillusioned with others, it is natural to look backward—to retrace your steps and try to figure out what went wrong. But sometimes, we go beyond remembering or evaluating history to denying or editing history in a desperate attempt to make sense of the pain. Even if this process provides a temporary resting place for our weary minds, the relief cannot be soul-deep because untruth cannot heal.

WHEN DISILLUSIONED WITH GOD'S PEOPLE, RESIST REVISIONISM.

To revise simply means to reexamine. *Revisionism*, however, describes a "departure from [an] original interpretation."[1] Departures are fine and even healthy *when* they are architected by the emergence of new, indisputable facts. However, when we are disillusioned, it is extremely easy to fall into a hurt-fueled (instead of fact-fueled) form of revisionism in which we rewrite the past in order to make sense of the present. Such efforts can sound something like this:

They must have had this planned from the very start.

I thought they loved me, but there's no way that could have been true.

In the beginning it seemed like a miracle, but it really was just a mistake.

I was sure that (fill-in-the-blank) was God's will, but based on how it ended, clearly I was wrong.

The last two lines could have come straight from my journals.

I felt awkward and awful. Wishing that invisibility were a genuine spiritual gift, I whispered, *"Lord, I should have said no from the very beginning. It would have saved others so much money and disappointment."*

The context was my first published book. How it came into being was, well, miraculous.

Ten years into our marriage, Barry and I turned our most requested teaching into a Bible study. Holding it in our hands was a pretty fabulous moment. But that was that. I did not think of myself as a writer, let alone an author. After all, a rather large chasm exists between someone saying, "I like to write," and others saying, "And we want to read!"

Consequently, publishing a book was nowhere on my radar when, after speaking at a church, a woman approached me and asked if I liked to write. Thinking of how much I enjoyed journaling, I said, "Oh yes! I love writing. It's so relaxing."

"Well," she replied, handing me a business card, "if you write like you speak, I'd like to talk with you further."

We shook hands, said goodbye, and I turned to greet the next kind soul who was waiting to talk with me. Once home, I pulled out the business card and was shocked to read, "Terri Gibbs, Vice President of

Acquisitions, JCountryman Division, Thomas Nelson." *What?!* Within two weeks, a book contract was on my desk!

The next few months were a wonderful whirlwind. Terri and her team asked me to provide the content for a beautiful devotional book they had crafted. The book's pages were gilded with silver, and the padded teal cover featured a single daisy in a simple vase with the title *Pure Joy*. The publisher flew me out to meet their incredible cast of sales reps and announced to the world that they had discovered "a female Max Lucado."

Bookstores shared their hope, and the first-quarter sales were impressive enough to risk signing me for another project. And then, most of the books that had been ordered *were returned to the publisher's warehouse*, unsold and unwanted. The beauty of the book could not offset how unknown I was as an author.

It felt terrible, like some dreadful combination of sadness, embarrassment, and regret. Terri and her team had risked so much for so little return, and, though she never said anything but kind words to me, I was beating myself up enough for the whole publishing house. *God, forgive me*, I cried. *Was it pride? Is that why I said yes? I'm so sorry. I thought I was being blessed by a miracle. But in reality, I was just making a big mess.*

This is revisionism. And this is what we must resist when disillusioned. Lies have no healing power. Yet how often do we go back and change the facts? How often do we spin the beginning to fabricate some sort of pseudo-peace about the end?

Deception cannot resolve disillusionment.

What was, was.

What is, is.

And in between what was and what is, is a powerful player called free will.

People change. Circumstances get rearranged. And God rarely draws in straight lines.

My revisionism brought me no relief. Nothing really did until a few years later when reality challenged my rewrite of history. The original story came to me verbally, but while writing this book I received an unrequested firsthand account in the mail. The sender had no idea that I was working on a manuscript, let alone planning to recount my first publishing experience. The following excerpt is shared from two beautiful, handwritten pages with the sender's permission:

> In the summer of 2004, when I should have been planning my precious daughter Kara's third birthday party, instead I stood over her tiny grave with a broken heart and a faith I felt sure was fractured beyond repair. That fall, I received a phone call that a lady from church was unable to attend a ladies' retreat and had donated her spot to me. Still very raw, I reluctantly agreed to attend. When I arrived and saw the book table at the back of the room, a book title jumped out at me. *Pure Joy*—that is the meaning of Kara Kathleen from the Greek word "chara" meaning "joy" and Kathleen which means "pure." These words are on Kara's headstone, and it was like God was letting me know He brought me there for a divine purpose, and that retreat, where you spoke, was the beginning of the mending process God was bringing to my heart and my faith.[2]

Well, then. I guess *Pure Joy* was a miracle after all! If only for this beautiful soul, everything, including the disappointment, was worth it.

When disillusioned, remember that painful endings do not have the authority to void miraculous beginnings. Resist the urge to make sense of the night through revisionism. An unresolved mystery is far safer for our souls than anesthetizing our minds with untruth.

Chapter 48

. . .

THE "SHOW ME"
STATE

There is an old saying that states, "It takes two to tango." The idiom was first coined in a song written in 1952 by Al Hoffman and Dick Manning. Thirty years later, the phrase was popularized by President Ronald Reagan when he used it to describe a matter of international relations.[1]

The tango is a partner dance.

There is no such thing as a solo tango.

A tango is not a tango unless it is a duo.

The phrase is used to describe something that cannot be done *alone*. When used in reference to an interpersonal conflict, "It takes two to tango" implies that both sides contributed to the problem.

Though the concept makes some sense, I question its absolute accuracy. Yes, by definition, interpersonal conflict requires more than one person. But that does not mean that all parties actively, let alone equally, joined in the dance. I have met more than a few people over the years who are quite skilled at creating relational drama all by themselves.

But even then—when to the best of our knowledge the only thing we have done to contribute to interpersonal pain is breathe—the fact remains that we are still imperfect and in-process. Even if we have not sinned against the other person in the conflict, we still have sin within us.

WHEN DISILLUSIONED WITH GOD'S PEOPLE, STAY TEACHABLE.

Every disillusionment contains within it the opportunity for hearts and love to be purified by God. But in order for that to happen, we must work to remain teachable when wronged and humble when in the right. And that is a very difficult thing to do. It requires our sincere cries of "But it's so unjust!" to rise and harmonize with Jesus' night cry of "Not my will, but yours be done" (Luke 22:42).

Of course it is not just.

How can it be?

This is not heaven.

Please know that my goal here is a reality check, not a guilt trip. (If you naturally tend to assume that everything is your fault, please apply this principle with caution.) Neither is my intention to register a vote for passivity. By all means, continue "to act justly" (Micah 6:8).

This encouragement to remain teachable when disillusioned with God's people is based in certainty that God does not waste anything here on earth. He will bring you "treasures of darkness" (Isaiah 45:3) in even the most unjust interpersonal pain as you keep choosing to follow Him through the night.

A while back, something that hardly ever happens to me happened twice within twenty-four hours. Two individuals, who did not know each other and had no idea what was going on in my life, reached out to say that God had impressed a Scripture on their hearts for me. Each person then proceeded to share the *exact* same passage—Joel 2:23-27—with an emphasis on verse 25, which reads, "I will repay you for the years the locusts have eaten."

Wow, well, that's something, I thought. *Evidently, God is going to return to me all that this unjust situation has stolen!* But then I sensed the Holy Spirit challenging me to read the entire story to understand the verses in context.

Joel is a fascinating book, but one aspect in particular stood out to me at that time. An enemy had come against God's people, and though the onslaught was extreme, God's call for His people was to repent (see Joel 1:13; 2:12). What He asked of them in the middle of the mess was teachability. He wanted them to learn to pay attention to their own hearts, as opposed to inspecting and dissecting the hearts of their enemies. God was using the crisis to purify His people and reveal His character: "Rend your heart and not your garments. Return to the LORD your God, for he is gracious and compassionate, slow to anger and abounding in love, and he relents from sending calamity" (Joel 2:13).

This was sobering.

Applying the principle to my own situation, my perspective began to shift from waiting to be vindicated to remembering that I too was vulnerable to sin—from focusing on what they had done to asking what I needed to do.

Yes, something had come against me. Yes, it seemed way out of proportion and extreme. To my knowledge, my own choices had not started it. To my frustration, my best words could not stop it.

But my assignment in the midst of it was neither to be indignant about the injustice nor to moan about the mess. My assignment was to remain teachable and attend to the sin that the crisis was bringing to the surface of my life.

With God's patience, my heart softened, and I became ready to learn. By God's grace, my prayer shifted from "Lord, show them!" to "Lord, show me." In short, God's kindness led me to repentance (see Romans 2:4), and remaining teachable helped purify my love.

Chapter 49

...

FROM ABOVE

One of the reasons our ability to love grows stronger through every cycle of disillusionment with God's people is because, as we lose illusions, our choice to keep loving occurs in the context *of greater accuracy.*

It is one thing to love the community of faith when we think it is perfect. It is quite another thing to love the community of faith when we know it is not. As we remain committed to the body of Christ *as it really is,* our love evolves from a gas to a solid, from something serendipitous to something sublime.

WHEN DISILLUSIONED WITH GOD'S PEOPLE, LOVE IN REALITY.

When disillusioned with other Jesus-followers, we have the opportunity to love them for who they actually are as opposed to who we thought they were or who we think they should be. This is where Jesus' command "As I have loved you, so you must love one another" (John 13:34) gets real.

Sometimes we snag on this verse, worried that it means we have to stay in a job regardless of how badly we are treated or we have to remain in a relationship regardless of how sickly it becomes. But as noted earlier, John 13:34 is not about going passive in the face of dysfunction. It is a call to follow Jesus' example in the face of reality. This is not about the spineless endorsement of everything done under the sun but the willful choice to love as Jesus loved.

Jesus loved the disciples *accurately*. He knew who they really were, but His love was not sourced in their behavior. Then and now, Jesus' love flows *from above*. This is how we can love people we do not like. This is how we can love someone even when we hope that we do not have to interact with them. We draw from God's above love and think to ourselves, *Okay, you are not at all who I thought you were. But we are both part of God's family. He loves you, so I'm going to keep trying until we see Him face-to-face.*

How?

By accepting the reality of who they are instead of punishing them emotionally for who they are not.

By, in the words of Saint Augustine, choosing again and again to forgive rather than allowing our enemies to be "held in hatred, lest . . . there be two bad men."[1]

By choosing to love, not because someone has earned it, but out of respect for our shared heavenly Father.

(And by remembering that someone, somewhere, is probably trying to do all the above for us.)

Loving in reality is powerful. This is the type of love I think our ultimate Realist, Jesus, had in mind when He said, "By this all men will know that you are my disciples, if you love one another" (John 13:35).

Many of us instinctively look to our emotions to confirm whether or not we are loving. But surely, Jesus, in His teachings and His example, was referencing not the *feeling* of love but the *choice* to love.

When we think of love as more of a feeling than a choice, it is virtually impossible to love in reality. Because, frankly, there are some souls we may never feel love for this side of heaven. Even then—when the feeling of love is lagging way, way behind our choice to love—though uncomfortable, it is sustainable.

We can do this.

You can do this.

Because God has already done this for us.

One of the first times God called me to *choose to love* even though I *felt nothing of love* was when an unshared expectation erupted among God's people, and I was swept downhill in the burn.

I can laugh (a little bit) now looking back on the sheer madness of it all, but at the time, it was not remotely funny. Shifting to an earlier metaphor, not only had I been unknowingly drafted into a tango, but I had no clue there had even been a dance until it was all over and I was summoned to the floor for critique. *Wait!* I protested in dismay. *When did the music begin? When did the doors even open? How can I be punished for not showing up for something that I didn't even know was happening?*

It was a ridiculous, illogical mess. And my feelings of love for those involved were among the many casualties of the conflict. Yet Jesus' call to "love one another" remained. *You'll have to mentor me through this,* I prayed. *I don't know how to love under these circumstances.*

In response, Jesus cautioned me to avoid two other types of "love": love that is imaginary and love that is mercenary.

Imaginary love is when we try to bring our feelings up to speed by lying to ourselves about the person or persons with whom we are disillusioned.

They aren't so bad. They didn't mean it.

They won't do it again. I'm sure they've changed.

Besides, it was all my fault. I brought this on myself.

Imaginary love is a near opposite of loving in reality. Any good feelings the fabrication of illusions may summon are simply a setup for more disillusionment. Just as we must face our own sins and stumblings, we cannot erase others' sins and stumblings.

The second type of love God called me to avoid was mercenary. To be mercenary is to be motivated "by self-interest or the pursuit of personal gain."[2] Sometimes we love to alter others or exonerate ourselves. Though being loved is transformational, the type of love that opens the door to transformation is not transactional. In other words, choosing to love in reality means loving to give, not loving to get.

So, when the feeling of love fails us in the night, let us choose to love in reality. Not by repainting the other as perfect. Nor by loving so that they will change their mind. But by following Jesus' very clear example: "We love because he first loved us" (1 John 4:19).

Chapter 50

· · ·

FORTY-FOUR
CHAPTERS PAST BAIL

Further complicating our understanding and application of Jesus' "love one another" in the community of faith is our tendency to treat *love* as a synonym for *trust*. These words are not interchangeable in the Scriptures.

An entire book could be devoted to this contrast. Even though both *love* and *trust* can be used as nouns, 1 John 4:16 states that God is not trust, but love. Love is something different from trust. Love is *other*. As mentioned in the last chapter, love is *from above*.

In the roughly sixty "one another" and "each other" New Testament verses that instruct us on life together, we are told to love one another well over a dozen times, yet we are not told to trust each other even once.

Granted, there are plenty of other admonitions that will keep us busy for the rest of our days. We are encouraged *to* honor, accept, instruct, greet, wait for, be devoted to, wash the feet of, serve, carry, be patient with, have equal concern for, be kind and compassionate toward, speak to, submit to, encourage, build up, spur on, confess our sins to, pray for, offer hospitality to, be humble toward, and live at peace and harmony with one another. And we are told *not to* pass judgment on, bite, devour, destroy, envy, grumble against, slander, provoke, be conceited toward, or lie to one another.

But unlike the call to "love one another" (which sounds repeatedly throughout the New Testament), trusting one another is not commanded or even suggested. It does not make the list as either a *do* or a *don't*. Trust is a different kind of thing altogether.

> Love is something *given*. Trust is something *earned*.
>
> Love is about *generosity*. Trust is about *safety*.
>
> Treating the two as synonyms can be disastrous.

The dysfunction that has been perpetuated under the banner of "If you love me, then you'll trust me" is appalling. You can do either without the other. You can trust a surgeon without loving them. And you can love a relative without trusting them.

Distinguishing between love and trust is an essential skill for navigating the troubled waters of disillusionment within the family of God, especially when the severity of interpersonal conflict and tension escalates to levels beyond human resolution.

In my early twenties, I would have dismissed that phrase—"beyond human resolution"—as pure pessimism. I remember thinking, *Sure, this is hard. But since we all love Jesus, resolution is only a few conversations away. We just need to keep talking. Once we understand each other's hearts more clearly, all will be well once again.*

Life soon schooled me otherwise. And when it did, the next principle became a lifesaver.

WHEN DISILLUSIONED WITH GOD'S PEOPLE,
NOTICE IF YOUR SHIELD STARTS SLIPPING.

A sage minister once graced me with unsolicited advice. We met at her church after I had just said yes to a new opportunity. Knowing more about the backstory than I would discern for years, she saw an enormous interpersonal storm on my horizon before I even noticed a cloud. Invited into her office, I was honored to have time with her but surprised by what she wanted to say.

"Alicia, I think you are fantastic. But not everyone is going to like you. In fact, there are two types of people who really will not like you . . ." She then proceeded to share her (what later would be revealed as *spot-on*) concerns.

"Really?" I said, oblivious. "Honestly, this is an area I feel really blessed in. I seem to get along with just about everyone."

She smiled and nodded. "Well, if God ever calls you to serve with these types of people, He will place a shield over your heart to protect you. But if that shield ever starts to fall, I want you to remember this conversation and give yourself permission to look for a way out."

I rarely use this word, but her counsel was prophetic. A few short years later, I finally grasped what it felt like for the shield to start slipping.

King David understood what this meant as well.

We make much in the Church of how David refused to lay a hand on "the Lord's anointed" (1 Samuel 26:9) and waited for God to remove Saul. While that is true, it is important to also remember that David did not *submit* to the Lord's anointed. If David had truly submitted to Saul, he would have stayed still when Saul—jealous, angry, and tormented—threw spears. (See 1 Samuel 18:10-11; 19:9-10).

But David did not surrender to Saul's sickness.

David did not self-martyr on Saul's spears.

David left.

Though he *loved* Saul—and would weep when he died—David could not *trust* Saul.

David is a great example for us when we are facing unresolvable conflicts within the faith family, not because he did not leave but because he never stopped loving. David stayed as long as he could. He used his gifts to try to bring Saul comfort. And I think leaving broke his heart. There was desperation, not arrogance, in David's departure. There was nothing cavalier about his exit from the palace.

Such unresolvable conflicts are most often (but not always) sourced in unrepentant sin and denied or unaided illness. David was not perfect, but there was nothing he could have done to dissolve Saul's jealousy or defuse Saul's rage. It was an internal fire that Saul let get out of control, and it burned all who came near him.

When we find ourselves in similar relationships, like David, we hope that "Saul" gets better. We pray for "Saul's" deliverance. But sometimes we need to hope and pray from a distance.

This is not bailing. In fact, this is forty-four chapters past bailing. This is when spiritual pain is sourced *in toxicity*, and when, like David, all our serving and all our worshiping cannot neutralize the poison.

I truly hope you never need this chapter.

But if you do, please remember: When the shield fell and Saul's spears were aimed at David's heart, David did leave Saul, but he never stopped loving Saul. When disillusioned with God's anointed, David remained committed to his Lord, his faith, and the family of God.

The choice to love, even when he had to leave, carried David (and can carry us) through the nights of disillusionment with the people of God.

Chapter 51

. . .

THE MAN
IN THE MIDDLE

It was baffling.

The situation was unpleasant, to say the least. But my emotional response was extreme. My chest was tight, and I could not sleep. Yes, the conflict was real, but it was not apocalyptic. *What on earth is going on, Lord?* I wondered.

Sometimes when our emotional responses are over the top (i.e., out of proportion to our circumstances), it is an indicator that the current pain is pressing on an older wound.

As I began to journal, this is exactly where God drew my attention. He showed me the similarities between this moderate conflict and one of the most painful experiences of disillusionment with God's people that I had ever known. Attending to that wound at the next layer on the spiral, I asked God to search my heart, repented of all He revealed, prayed through another round of forgiveness, and chose once again to love.

Then an image came to mind that reminded me of a showdown from an old Western movie. I saw myself facing off with someone at the proverbial twenty paces of distance. Our postures were adversarial, but we had no weapons in hand. Then I saw Jesus in between us, not in the middle, but right in front of the other person with His back toward me. I sensed His gentle voice saying, *Alicia, I have already absorbed 99.9% of their toxicity. What hit you was just the overspray.*

This had never occurred to me, but surely it was true. Jesus had been between us the entire time, no doubt absorbing more than I could ever imagine from us both.

What still reached me *was real*, and honestly, it felt like acid on my soul. But it was just the overspray of all Jesus had absorbed. Overwhelmed by this reality, I sensed one more whisper: *So, Alicia, will you fellowship with Me in My sufferings?*

And there it was—the perspective I needed to survive spiritual pain that came from within the family of God.

When we are disillusioned, it can seem as though God has His back to us. But spiritually, what is really happening is that God is facing off what has come against us. He is the Man in the middle of all our interpersonal pain in the faith family. And every loss of an illusion and every gain of a reality is actually an opportunity to fellowship with Him, our Savior and First Love.

Have you ever been disillusioned with the people of God? Have you ever lost illusions and gained reality about life together as a community of faith? Have you ever felt lost in a night of interpersonal pain?

If so . . .

Be slow to assume that sin is the source.

Humbly acknowledge that your strengths might have shadows.

Learn to listen generously.

Articulate your expectations.

Cultivate mental flexibility.

Know when it is not your cow.

Speak to heal, not to harm.

Resist revisionism.

Stay teachable.

Love in reality.

And notice if your shield starts slipping.

As we fix our eyes on the Man in the middle, He will show us the way.

When I first began studying interpersonal disillusionment from Genesis to Revelation, it was obvious that the Scriptures contained far more examples of *conflict* than of *conflict resolution*. Clearly, something stronger than our skills holds us together as the family of God, generation after generation. Though I pray that these tools will help you, our true hope is in something more powerful, present, and precious than all our best efforts combined.

Our true hope is not the family of God; it is the God of the family.

What happened between Barnabas and Paul is, perhaps, the best-known early church example of disillusionment between two sincere Jesus-followers. The same strength that initiated their friendship ultimately contributed to their rift. Their powerful partnership began because Barnabas was willing to take a risk on Paul (see Acts 9:26-28). And the dissolution of that partnership—their "sharp disagreement"—occurred when Barnabas was willing to take a risk on Mark (see Acts 15:36-41).

Though this story would have made an excellent example for the chapter on strength shadows, I intentionally reserved it for now. Why? To position our true hope when disillusioned *higher than ourselves*.

Yes, Barnabas and Paul parted ways.

And God went with Paul.

And God went with Barnabas.

Because they were both fully right and righteous? Doubtful. Our perfection has never been the prerequisite for God's companionship.

His love is what holds us together. As we commit to God's upward pull of love through disillusionment, we remain connected by God's Spirit even if our earthly paths diverge.

Spiritual pain in the family is an age-old problem. And for God, it was an anticipated problem. Recalling a statement from an earlier chapter, we are different people from different places with different pasts, pains, and personalities. Add to that mix different cultures and generations, and it is a miracle that we ever understand each other at all.

Yet Jesus calls us all together and prays, "Father, may they be one."

> My prayer is not for them alone. I pray also for those who will believe in me through their message, that all of them may be one, Father, just as you are in me and I am in you. May they also be in us so that the world may believe that you have sent me. I have given them the glory that you gave me, that they may be one as we are one: I in them and you in me. May they be brought to complete unity to let the world know that you sent me and have loved them even as you have loved me.
> JOHN 17:20-23

What on earth does *that* mean?

Our infinitely creative God intentionally made us infinitely different. Those differences guarantee disillusionment before sin even enters the room. So *being one* cannot be on hold, awaiting some utopian calm sourced in sameness. Surely, what *being one* is awaiting is the presence of devotion and commitment, not the absence of difference and conflict.

Within our shared painful gaining of reality, may God strengthen us to choose again and again to remain devoted to Jesus and, *through Jesus*, committed to the other souls gathered around His table.

Not for commitment's sake.

Not for our own sake.

But for Christ's sake.

Because He is committed to us.

And He has committed us to one another.

We are His body on this earth.

In the day and through the night.

Chapter 52

. . .

CONCLUSION

In the night—in the midst of spiritual pain—although understanding may elude us, God's presence accompanies us, always pulling us upward into His love. The *how* of not bailing—the *how* of staying committed when disillusioned with God, ourselves, and one another—is strenuous but not mysterious. We try to complicate that *how*, but Jesus keeps it quite simple.

In the night, as in the day, He simply says, "Follow Me."

Even when in pain?

Yes, my friend, *especially* when in pain.

Following Jesus is the self-sustaining core of commitment and the not-so-cryptic key to spiritual growth through disillusionment. Every time you choose to follow Jesus in the night, your faith grows and you build momentum to keep following Him in the days (and decades) to come.

Granted, it is hard to follow someone when we can neither see (because of the darkness) nor imagine where they are going (because we have never been there before). But I have had to follow others under similar circumstances, and my guess is you have too.

When driving behind a friend, following them with no clue as to where they are going, we know what to do:

We stay close to keep them in our sight.

We watch carefully to mirror their movements.

And we quickly address anything that might block our clear view.

This is doable. Following is possible. And yes, we would prefer Jesus (and our friend) to just give us an address so that we can type it into a GPS and get there on our own. But Jesus tends to be rather minimalistic when it comes to directions.

Instead, He calls us *to follow*.

Because faith *is relational*.

Thankfully, we are not the first generation to follow Jesus at night.

How to follow Jesus was a topic of conversation between Jesus and His very first disciples. Right before His arrest, Jesus revealed to Peter that he was about to deny Jesus three times (i.e., dark days are ahead). Immediately afterward, Jesus told them to "not let [their] hearts be troubled" (John 14:1) and then assured them that He was going away to prepare a place for them in His Father's house.

> "If I go and prepare a place for you, I will come back and take you to be with me that you also may be where I am. You know the way to the place where I am going." Thomas said to him, "Lord, we don't know where you are going, so how can we know the way?" Jesus answered, "I am the way and the truth and the life. No one comes to the Father except through me."
>
> JOHN 14:3-6

Thomas, like us, wanted directions. And Jesus gave him all the direction he would ever need: *Himself.*

Not latitude or longitude, but love.

Follow Jesus, and you *will* find your way Home.

I look forward to meeting you there, if not before. And I pray that, by God's grace, these words will have somehow helped you commit again, and again, and again, and again through disillusionment to the upward pull of God's love. As Gerald G. May has noted, "The process just keeps going on. . . . It just keeps deepening, revealing more and more intimate layers of freedom for love."[1]

To finish the story I began with, sitting on that park bench so many years ago, it never occurred to me that my night was leading me into greater "freedom for love." The spiritual pain was overwhelming. I feared that I had failed my faith and that my faith was about to fail me. Jesus was my world. And I could not shake the feeling that my world was caving in. I had run out of words and was running out of hope.

Then God brought to my mind a true story I recently had heard about a father and his son. The little boy loved holding his daddy's hand, but since his own hand was so small, he could only grip his daddy's pinkie. So, he gripped that pinkie with all his might. The dad would smile and deliberately secure his own thumb and the rest of his fingers firmly around his son's wrist.

One day as they were crossing a parking lot hand in hand, a pickup truck raced out of control around a corner and came straight toward them. In fear, the little boy did what he thought he never would do: he let go of his daddy's hand. The father, whose grip was still tightly around his son's wrist, pulled the little boy up out of the truck's path and into safety.

The boy was grateful but stunned. All along, he had been certain that it was *his* strength that kept his dad close. It was only when in fear he let go of his dad's hand that he found out otherwise. It took a time of helplessness to learn that he had always been in his father's grip.[2]

When I first heard that story, it did not occur to me that it might have relevance for my faith. That day in the park, however, the story became life to me. Collapsing on the picnic table, I released my fear *of spiritual failure*.

Wherever loss led me, deep within I somehow knew that Jesus would still be there. Too exhausted mentally and emotionally to grip faith myself, I discovered that Another—the focus of my faith—had always been gripping me. God reminded me that faith was not my creation. He was "the author and perfecter" of my faith (Hebrews 12:2). And His breath would sustain my faith even when my mind could not and my emotions would not.

Through the friend of disillusionment, I lost the illusion of a self-created faith and gained the reality of a faith-imparting God. The picnic table became an altar as my fear gave way to something far more satisfying than answers: the living, ever-giving love of God. He would, in the words of King David, "keep my lamp burning" (Psalm 18:28). Which meant that I never, ever needed to be afraid when the lights went out.

As Oswald Chambers said, "Faith in God is a terrific venture in the dark."[3]

Indeed.

What a relief! Our nights are normal.

Appendix A

• • •

OBJECTIONS

Named after its thesis statement, my doctoral dissertation was entitled "Disillusionment: An Unexpected Friend of Spiritual Formation." A dissertation often includes an identification of objections to its thesis. That process (of identifying and responding to objections in my dissertation) strengthened the framework I presented in this book.

For any who might find that defense process helpful, five objections to my claim that disillusionment is an unexpected friend of spiritual formation are excerpted below from my dissertation. The first is *fundamental*, the second is *definitional*, and the remaining three are *primary*.

OBJECTION ONE:

There Is No God with Whom to Become Disillusioned.

Starting points matter. Those who begin with a starting point of atheism consider belief in the existence of God to be an illusion and, therefore, view disillusionment as a means of dissing religious beliefs entirely. As a former atheist, this objection is familiar. As a current Jesus-follower, this objection cannot be countered without entering into a discussion of proofs for the existence and nonexistence of God, which is well beyond the scope of this book. Therefore, I acknowledge the objection that, from a nontheist's perspective, committing to love God through the experience of disillusionment is considered a step backward in psychological and social evolution.

OBJECTION TWO:

Claiming That Disillusionment Is a Friend Places a Tool in the Hands of Oppressors.

Those who suffer are not always disillusioned. Disillusionment, defined in this book as the act of removing false spiritual ideas, is not synonymous with suffering. However, the relationship between disillusionment and suffering is too porous to exempt the concept of disillusionment from being misused in the same way that the concept of suffering has been misused, hence the description of this objection as definitional. Some understandably will hesitate to accept the claim that disillusionment is a friend of spiritual formation because they fear that such a claim could be used as a tool of oppression. As feminist theologian Deanna A. Thompson asserts,

> From blaming the Jews for Jesus' death, to the Crusades, to invoking the cross as justification for the silent suffering of women, Christianity must confront the ways in which its theology and resulting practices glorify and even cause undeserved suffering.[1]

> No doctrine is more problematic, and no symbol more potentially destructive to women and other marginalized persons, than the doctrine of Christology and the symbol of the cross.[2]

"Suffer," the oppressor mocks. "It is good for your soul." Were I able to universally redeem disillusionment as a concept, some distance from this objection could be purchased. However, given the certainty that disillusionment will continue to be viewed by many as a form of suffering and a cross to bear, this objection stands.

Greed and power defile holy spaces. Since I view disillusionment as a holy space, with sadness I accept that disillusionment cannot escape the potential of such defilement. However, my confidence in defining disillusionment in terms of losing illusions and gaining realities is that the disillusioned will be interiorly and interpersonally strengthened. Illusions are tools of oppression. Let us celebrate their loss. Reality is a champion of interior freedom and social change. Let us celebrate its gain.

OBJECTION THREE:

Faith Is a Proclamation of the Positive. Therefore, Treating Disillusionment as an Unexpected Friend Encourages Negative Thinking.

This first of three primary objections to be considered is popular but perhaps not academic. In other words, though I encountered no scholars who voiced this objection, one stroll through a Christian bookstore testifies to its popular presence. This objection holds that since "faith is being sure of what we hope for and certain of what we do not see" (Hebrews 11:1), and since "the tongue has the power of life and death" (Proverbs 18:21), we should only verbalize positive thoughts and perspectives. For example, regardless of how you actually feel, speaking in faith that you are healthy confesses, and consequently brings into existence, health in your body.

Understandably, such a perspective would avoid most words that begin with *dis-*, including disease, disability, discouragement, and disillusionment. Philip Yancey discusses this objection in *Disappointment with God*:

> Some Christians, I know, would reject the phrase "disappointment with God" out of hand. Such a notion is all wrong, they say. Jesus promised that faith the size of a grain of mustard seed can move mountains; that anything can happen if two or three gather together in prayer. The Christian life is a life of victory and triumph. God wants us happy, healthy, and prosperous, and *any* other state simply indicates a lack of faith.[3]

A visit to a church that held this view contributed to Yancey's decision to write his classic book. In this church, parents were encouraged to proclaim the positive as an act of believing-faith for their sick children's healing.

As they buried their children, "they blame[d] themselves for weak faith. Meanwhile, the tombstones multiply."[4]

Without hesitation, I agree that words are powerful and that faith is the substance of things hoped for. However, I disagree with this objection's understanding of *faith-filled* speech. In the above example, I contend that *faith-filled speech* manifested as a form of psychological denial and intentional, albeit benevolent, alignment with untruth. If faith-filled speech means positivity over reality, then the writer of Hebrews as well as every writer in the biblical canon is guilty of faithless negativity, for the Scriptures are filled with expressions of despair, accounts of failure, and chronicles of pain. Theologian Julian Norris Hartt adds:

> We people of the Church feel impelled to convert the Church into a cheering-squad; and we go about with our own patented short-run assurances and nostrums. . . . Perhaps the people of this age do not quite know that the people of the Church are largely with them in the land of deep confusion and comprehensive fears. Well, let the fact be known. Our willingness to confess that we too have put feet upon the ice-bound shores of despair identifies us wholly with them. Our confession that God in Jesus Christ has found us there and has wrought resurrection, identifies us as at one with him, in hope and in love.[5]

Faith is the overflow of humility, not positivity. Faith is a mysterious muscle that, according to New Testament writers, is strengthened through trials and life's negatives.[6] Jesus' example on the cross of uttering, "My God, why have you forsaken me?"[7] and "Father, into your hands I commit my spirit"[8] demonstrate that "negative" emotions and biblical faith coexist in committed souls. As Peter L. Steinke states, "Those who insist on a 'pure' faith unstained by human emotionality make the denial of reality a condition of faith."[9]

Disillusionment is not the abandonment of faith-filled speech, but rather the movement of faith toward what is real.

OBJECTION FOUR:

Suicide Is the Ultimate Manifestation of Disillusionment.
Therefore, Disillusionment Should Be Viewed As an Enemy, Not a
Friend, of Spiritual Formation.

This objection negates the friendship of disillusionment based upon the
premise that suicide is an outcome of disillusionment: How can disillusionment be a friend of spiritual formation when its presence can trig-
ger the tragedy of suicide?[10] My response to this objection addresses the
soundness of its underlying premise.

Psychiatrist Anthony Reading in *Hope and Despair: How Perceptions of
the Future Shape Human Behavior* describes several mental states as represented in the following table.

Disillusioned	The result of expecting "either too much or too little of themselves or the world."[11]
Sadness and unhappiness	These are "*current-state* emotions that indicate that things are not presently going as we would like. . . . *Sadness*, a normal part of everyday living, is characterized by a mildly depressed mood without any change in our future hopes or expectations."[12]
Grief and depression	"*Prospective* emotions signifying to us that some or all of our future expectations are no longer attainable and prompting us to review the assumptions on which they were based."[13]
	"Grief is a temporary, self-healing response to a specific loss, such as occurs with death, divorce, or abandonment. It can also be triggered by the loss of material possessions or important beliefs."[14]
	"Grief signifies the loss of a circumscribed source of expectations which temporarily disturbs our everyday activities, while depression involves a more pervasive loss of hoped-for eventualities which disrupts our sense of well-being so greatly that we no longer know what to do or where to turn."[15]
Suicide[16]	"Represents the ultimate expression of despair, the absolute inability to foresee a tolerable future for oneself."[17]

For Reading, disillusionment is the experience of having unrealistic expectations (i.e., illusions) shattered by reality. Suicide, however, is prompted not by unmet expectations but by the absence of any hope-filled expectations.

What Reading calls sadness and unhappiness, Rabbi Elie Kaplan Spitz—who speaks of despair on a continuum—refers to as common depression, an experience which "occurs during day-to-day living in the space between contentment and angst, between expectations met and disappointments encountered."[18] Related to Spitz's despair is Hegel's "ascetic unhappy consciousness" and Kierkegaard's description of a "demonic" form of despair, which, if unresolved by faith, places "suicide [as] the danger nearest to him."[19]

Medical doctor Abraham J. Twerski explains that the despair that can lead to suicide is a "feeling [of being] utterly useless [which] goes beyond pain, resulting in a total numbness. The absence of all feeling puts one's very existence into question. A person in despair may feel that there is no place for him or her on the planet Earth."[20]

Rabbi Spitz writes both as a counselor and as one intimately familiar with theological despair.[21] Spitz, who illustrates his teaching with personal experiences of clinical depression and suicidal thoughts, states with humility, "I am aware that each one of us is capable of spiraling into darkness, of undergoing the emotional unraveling that leads to chaos. I understand that we cannot explain our emotions with our intellect."[22] He adds, "The truth is that although suffering is an inevitable part of the human condition, even in the face of such suffering we have the power to choose."[23] The challenge is to "be open to messages of hope, to form an identity of purpose, and to perceive the goodness in the world" as opposed to experiencing "our struggles as burdens, identifying as victims in a world of sorrow," which leads us to "compromise the capacity of our spirits to bear weight."[24]

Is suicide the outcome of disillusionment? As demonstrated above, psychologists and psychiatrists concur that suicide is the manifestation not of disillusionment as the loss of illusions, but of extreme despair as the loss of hope. I assert that disillusionment—the act of removing false ideas—does not cause suicide in the same way that a road does not cause a fatality. Disillusionment and roads are both paths: their navigation is in the hands of those who tread them, and their surfaces are often made more slippery by elements beyond the treader's control.

OBJECTION FIVE:

Disillusionment Is Self-Imposed. Therefore, It Can Be Avoided by Right Thinking.

Gene Edward Veith, provost and professor of literature at Patrick Henry College, views disillusionment as a state experienced by those who have not yet understood a key Christian doctrine. He believes, "It should not be possible for Christians to be disillusioned. We should have no illusions in the first place. Our faith is in Jesus Christ alone."[25] Describing a pattern he has often observed in others' descent into disillusionment, Veith observes the following:

> Many people who lose their intellectual grip on their faith do so because they become disillusioned. . . . They become aware of some of the shameful parts of the history of the Church. . . . Or, what can be even more devastating, they have had a bad experience in their own church. . . . They start assuming that the great doctrines of the faith, including the Incarnation and the Redemption, are nothing more than mere dogmas of the Church. They drift further and further away, until their faith, which once may have been extremely ardent, dwindles to a memory.[26]

Veith proposes theology as a solution to disillusionment: "Christians must fully understand the doctrine of sin so that they themselves do not become disillusioned. Offenses will indeed come (Matthew 18:7). Christians must take care not to be devastated by them. The doctrine of sin should ensure that they have no illusions to lose."[27] A strong grasp of the doctrine of sin can, from Veith's perspective, immunize believers from disillusionment via "Christian realism," which, "tough-minded and compassionate at the same time, can give a Christian an illuminating perspective on all of life."[28] His logic progresses as follows: *if* one believes that all are sinners, *then* one will not be surprised when sinners sin; *therefore* one will not distance oneself from God as a response to unnecessary disappointment.

My response to this objection is threefold. First, though I agree that an understanding of the doctrine of sin is useful toward the development of more reasonable expectations of one another, I disagree with Veith's assertion that disillusionment with God can be preempted theologically by avoiding disillusionment with humans. Was Job disillusioned with people or with God? Was Solomon disillusioned with people or with God? On that park bench, was I disillusioned with people or with God?

Not all disillusionment is sourced in interpersonal pain. Even for spiritual disillusionment that is sourced in disillusionment with people, Veith's statement that we "should have no illusions" reveals an assumed premise that such a continually objective state is possible.

To be objective is to base decisions upon facts as opposed to feelings or opinions: to see things truly as they exist "outside of the mind."[29] Though one may be able to approach objectivity in certain areas, absolute objectivity is somewhat mythical.[30] Subjectivity—not objectivity—is our natural state as humans. As such, illusions—inaccurate ideas—are inevitable.

With regard to the painful loss of such illusions, Reading explains, "The various forms of sadness and despair that afflict our spirits and give us pause are, unfortunately, unavoidable parts of the human condition."[31] Rabbi Spitz adds that the "ancient heroes and healers from the Bible offer us comfort by demonstrating that despair is ancient and eternal."[32] Is it therefore realistic to assume that finite beings seeking to interact with and interpret an infinite God—and all that an infinite God has created—will instinctively do so accurately?

Second, I grant that in my description of disillusionment as inevitable, allowance must be made for the fact that not *all* disillusionment is inevitable. Allowing our expectations to be adjusted by wisdom gleaned from personal experience and the Spirit's mentoring can successfully dismiss some experiences of disillusionment with a preemptive acceptance of reality. Such is exemplified in a story recounted by Philip Yancey of a man named Douglas, whose life resembled that of a modern-day Job. When asked if he was disappointed with God, Douglas replied,

> I have learned to see beyond the physical reality in this world
> to the spiritual reality. We tend to think, "Life should be fair
> because God is fair." But God is not life. And if I confuse God
> with the physical reality of life—by expecting constant good
> health, for example—then I set myself up for a crashing dis-
> appointment. God's existence, even his love for me, does not
> depend on my good health.[33]

Expectations are powerful forces deserving of careful monitoring. Douglas was not disillusioned because he did not possess the expectation (i.e., illusion) that "life should be fair because God is fair." As referenced previously, psychiatrist Anthony Reading speaks of how those who "expected either too much or too little of themselves or the world . . . ended up being disillusioned and dispirited."[34] Un-critiqued expectations can create dangerous illusions, for, in the words of Screwtape, "Whatever men expect, they soon come to think they have a right to: the sense of disappointment can, with very little skill on our part, be turned into a sense of injury."[35] Therefore, I agree with Veith in part: some experiences of disillusionment can be self-imposed via un-critiqued expectations.

Third, though I agree that faith from the start is a reciprocal embrace by the Greater Reality that is God, I suggest that we awaken to God much as does a child to their mother. (Please note that the following

discussion also appears in chapter 7.) In other words, our grasp of reality is ever-evolving. If an infant could talk, they might say that "Mom is
milk," and perhaps later that "Mom is hands and eyes." Even when the
toddler could describe Mom head-to-toe as a distinct person, they would
still spend their life discovering—through interpreting and reinterpreting,
through hypothesis and correction or confirmation—Mom's inner being.
After Mom dies, the child would still be pondering the complex depths
of Mom and considering, in their own final breath, much of Mom as a
lovely mystery. Technically speaking, the infant's thought that "Mom is
milk" is an illusion: an inaccurate idea. Yet, in all its inaccuracy, "Mom is
milk" reflects the infant's healthy development. From birth to death, life
is a continual shedding of illusions.

In conclusion, I offer an example from the life of C. H. Spurgeon that
illustrates the inadequacy of right thinking as a deterrent for all disillusionment. Although Spurgeon suffered physically for decades, it was
the pain of the October 19, 1856, Royal Surrey Garden tragedy that
prompted the phrase "furnace of mental suffering" in his autobiography.[36]
Spurgeon was preaching that night to a crowd of over 10,000 when an
unknown voice cried, "Fire!" In the ensuing panic, seven people died,
and Spurgeon's anguish over the event cast a long and deep shadow over
his life.

By Veith's reasoning, Spurgeon's commitment to the doctrine of sin should
have sufficiently shielded him from excessive spiritual despair. Humans
are sinners, and sinners sin. Therefore, whether the Music Hall stampede
and resulting deaths were caused by intentional malice or fear-inspired
panic, Spurgeon should have had no illusions that such things could not
or would not occur. Few, however, would question Spurgeon's theological
thoughtfulness and perhaps even fewer would question the reality of his
mental and spiritual anguish following the experience. Historian Dr. Peter
J. Morden notes, "Following the disaster Spurgeon spoke of his thoughts
being like a 'case of knives' cutting his heart 'in pieces.' It was a time of
unrelenting 'misery' and 'darkness.'"[37]

Spurgeon spoke from his anguish in a sermon entitled "A Question for a Questioner" on Psalm 77:9:

> Pain of body, when it is continuous and severe, is exceedingly trying to our feeble spirits; but agony of soul is worse still. Give me the rack sooner than despair. . . . When Asaph had prayed for relief, and the relief did not come, the temptation came to him to ask, "Am I always to suffer? Will the Lord never relieve me? It is written, 'He healeth the broken in heart, and bindeth up their wounds'; has he ceased from that sacred surgery? 'Hath God forgotten to be gracious?'"[38]

In these words are heard the ache-spring of spiritual disillusionment. The variations are many, but the manifestation is similar: an illusion, an interrogative, a woeful wonder at reality's seeming misalignment of God's character and ways. The mind loses its footing in the incongruence. Through disillusionment, thinking and theology bow to, and then are reshaped by, God Himself.

Appendix B

• • •

OCCURRENCES OF *DISILLUSION* IN ENGLISH TRANSLATIONS OF THE BIBLE[1]

Verse	Version	Quotation (emphasis added)	Word Analysis
Ps. 7:14	NIV, 1978, 2011	"Whoever is pregnant with evil conceives trouble and gives birth to **disillusionment**."	שֶׁקֶר (*šě·qěr*): Deception, misleading falseness, i.e., a state or condition which is utterly false, and causes a mistaken belief.[2] *šě·qěr* appears 113x in the NIV and is most often translated as forms of *lie/lying* (52x), *false* (27x), and *deception* (12x).[3]
Isa. 20:5	Good News Trans., 1966, 1992	"Those who have put their trust in Ethiopia and have boasted about Egypt will be **disillusioned**, their hopes shattered."	חָתַת (*hā·tǎt*): Be dismayed, i.e., have a feeling of discouragement, implying fear and terror, and/or panic and confusion, as an extension of the shattering of an object.[4] NIV 1984 translates as "will be afraid."
Isa. 20:5	Expanded Bible, 2011	"People who looked to Cush for help [trusted/put hope in Cush] *will be afraid* [dismayed; **disillusioned**]."	Same as above.

Verse	Version	Quotation (emphasis added)	Word Analysis
Jer. 10:14	Good News Trans., 1966, 1992	"At the sight of this, people feel stupid and senseless; those who make idols are **disillusioned**, because the gods they make are false and lifeless."	בָּעַר (bā-'ār): Be senseless, i.e., to think and act as a fool.[5] NIV translates as "every goldsmith is **shamed** by his idols." bā-'ār appears 120x in the NIV and is translated with forms of *shame* 87x and *disgrace* 17x.[6]
Jer. 48:13	Good News Trans., 1966, 1992	"Then the Moabites will be **disillusioned** with their god Chemosh, just as the Israelites were **disillusioned** with Bethel, a god in whom they trusted."	בּוֹשׁ (bôš): Be ashamed, i.e., to have a painful feeling and emotional distress (sometimes to the point of despair) by having done something wrong, with an associative meaning of having the disapproval of those around them (Judg. 3:25; Jer. 14:4). Note: This wrong can refer to a social mistake or a serious sin.[7] NIV translates bôš in Jer. 48:13 as *ashamed*.
Jer. 51:17	Good News Trans., 1966, 1992	"At the sight of this, people feel stupid and senseless; those who make idols are **disillusioned** because the gods they make are false and lifeless."	See Jer. 10:14, above.
Hosea 9:3	The Message, 2002, 2018	"At this rate you'll not last long in God's land: Some of you are going to end up bankrupt in Egypt. Some of you will be **disillusioned** in Assyria."	NIV, ASV, RSV translation: "eat unclean food in Assyria." Peterson translates the outcome, whereas the text speaks of the means.

Appendix C

· · ·

A BRIEF ETYMOLOGY
OF DISILLUSIONMENT

The English language began to bubble up in the linguistic pool in the fifth century. But we have to wade through a thousand years of history in order to find the first known occurrence of any variation of *disillusionment*. *Disillusion* first appeared in a 1598 English translation of a Spanish romance novel by Jorge de Montemayor titled *Los siete libros de la Diana*: "What slights, what disillusions . . . have risen from such sorrows?"[1]

The second known occurrence of *disillusion* occurs 250 years later in Elizabeth Barrett Browning's reflections on her poem *Casa Guidi Windows*. Contemplating the discrepancy between the first and second part of her poem, which were written three years apart, Browning stated,

> Such discrepancy we are called to accept at every hour by the condition of our nature . . . the discrepancy between aspiration and performance, between faith and dis-illusion, between hope and fact.

> *O trusted, broken prophecy,*
> *O richest fortune sourly crost,*
> *Born for the future, to the future lost!*[2]

Whereas Montemayor used *disillusion* as a synonym for sorrow-inspired slights, Browning contrasted *disillusion* with faith. Even in its first appearances, the word seemed to capture a soul-deep sadness that challenged one's beliefs.

And then, almost fifteen hundred years after the emergence of the English language, we finally encounter the earliest known occurrence of the noun *disillusionment*. In 1856, in a travel magazine entitled *The Leisure Hour*, a guide wrote, "The first few days in Rome . . . must be a disappointment—a sort of *disillusionment*, if we may coin that term."[3]

(Thank you, *Leisure Hour*. Surely the coining was not great—or even accurate—news for Rome. But the word has been a true gift to us.)

Appendix D

. . .

A COMMENTARY ON RELATED TERMS AND CONCEPTS

The running table in chapter 4 is an inevitably incomplete summary of scholars consulted in this study,[1] listed chronologically by date of birth. What follows is a brief commentary on several of the terms that are most closely related to our theme of disillusionment.

One quick glance confirms the inclusion of both secular and religious thinkers in this summary. Without question, starting points matter. If one views God as an illusion, then spiritual disillusionment is a means of evolution by which God-concepts are relinquished. If one views God as real, then spiritual disillusionment is a means of growth by which God-concepts are refined. Since pure objectivity is mythical for humanity, the premises with which we start directly affect the conclusions with which we end.

Both perspectives are included because both perspectives have shaped our modern understanding of spiritual pain.

GENESIS, PSEUDO-DIONYSIUS, JOHN OF THE CROSS, AND MAY ON DARKNESS

The term that most consistently, through the centuries, overlaps with our working definition of disillusionment is *darkness*. Darkness is referenced innumerable times, starting with the first lines of the book of Genesis. In the beginning, "darkness was over the surface of the deep, and the Spirit of God was hovering over the waters" (Genesis 1:2).

God, evidently, sees quite well in the dark. Before humankind took a God-given breath, God and darkness were at home together on earth. As stated earlier, pre-Fall, pre-sin, and pre-humanity, darkness is one of the original inhabitants of earth. Fourteen chapters later, we find God at home again in a "thick and dreadful darkness" within which He makes a covenant with Abraham.[2]

Scripture and Christian literature through the ages have acknowledged the relationship between darkness and intimacy with God. Even today, darkness is used metaphorically for seasons in which reason stumbles so that our spirits may advance. Which is quite similar to how, in disillusionment, reason stumbles as false ideas are lost and new realities are gained.

In the sixth century, Pseudo-Dionysius spoke of a gift to spiritual formation which he called a darkness that outshines all brilliance.[3] This early teacher believed that such divine darkness revealed that intimacy with God was beyond the work of humanity. In other words, when the intellect cries for mercy, God answers by revealing a deeper measure—not of understanding, but love.

Eight centuries later, the anonymous author of *The Cloud of Unknowing* likewise wrote of

> darkness and this cloud [that] is, howsoever thou dost, betwixt thee and thy God, and letteth thee that thou mayest neither see Him clearly by light of understanding in thy reason, nor feel Him in sweetness of love in thine affection. And therefore shape thee to bide in this darkness as long as thou mayest, evermore crying after Him that thou lovest.[4]

Echoing the triad of divine darkness, the limits of human understanding, and the invitation to greater intimacy with God, *Dark Night of the Soul* and *The Ascent of Mount Carmel* were offered two centuries later by John of the Cross. According to John, love guides us through the darkness into union with God. As Gerald G. May summarizes, John's "dark night" is a "co-participation between God and person"[5] which "helps us become who we are created to be: lovers of God and one another."[6] Like Pseudo-Dionysius and the anonymous author of *The Cloud of Unknowing*, John taught that the path to greater love and spiritual insight often wended its way through darker seasons of mental anguish.

REITMAN, WALSH, PODMORE, YANCEY, JACOBSON, AND SPURGEON ON ECCLESIASTES AND JOB

As discussed in chapter 4, as an English word, *disillusion* appears a scarce seven times in four out of forty-plus English translations of the Bible. However, disillusionment as an experience is represented throughout the Scriptures, and perhaps most prominently through the words of Ecclesiastes and the story of Job.

The writer of Ecclesiastes (*Qoheleth* in the Hebrew), most probably Solomon, pens his despair over the meaninglessness of life on earth. James S. Reitman and Jerome T. Walsh both write insightfully regarding the source and outcome of Qoheleth's spiritual pain. Reitman notes that the Hebrew concept of disillusionment is carried in the original language of Ecclesiastes 5:17, which he translates, "All his days he eats in darkness and *is greatly disillusioned* in his sickness and anger."[7] Reitman states that the "concept of 'disillusionment' is conveyed by the root וְכָעַס but this is not obvious in most English translations."[8] From Reitman's perspective, the illusion lost by the writer is that of self-sufficiency: "Qoheleth's reflections are designed to leave self-sufficient readers with no hope of fulfilling their foolish and presumptuous schemes."[9] In both Job and Ecclesiastes, Reitman sees compelling examples of the rocky journey from self-reliance to wisdom.[10] Reitman explains: "For those readers who finally 'get' the ultimate futility of self-sufficiency, the rhetorical goal in both books is *to provoke sufficient disillusionment* that they might *relinquish self-reliant strategies for meaning, fear God, accept their God-given portion in life, and invest wisely in God's ongoing redemptive purpose.*"[11]

Jerome T. Walsh identifies a different illusion lost in Ecclesiastes: the expectation that genuine spirituality will be vibrant spirituality. In a thought-provoking article entitled "Despair as a Theological Virtue," Walsh addresses this agonizing form of disillusionment. After asserting that the tenets of Christianity still do not answer the core questions of Ecclesiastes, Walsh borrows the name *Qoheleth* to refer to the hidden souls in the Church who have chosen faithfulness to a God they do not feel. Their "dryness in prayer and sense of divine-absence" isolate them, and from Walsh's perspective, the untraditional spirituality of the author of Ecclesiastes can comfort them, for "to support another traveler in the darkness and from the darkness, to share one's own growing trust of darkness, is to offer, like Qoheleth himself, the consolation of companionship if not of explanation."[12] Though most are familiar with what Simon Podmore so eloquently describes as faith that "feel[s] at a melancholy distance from its savior,"[13] Walsh gives voice to the souls for whom felt distance is normative, souls for whom commitment to and intimacy with God is real, but not felt.

For insight into the disillusionment of Job, we turn to the writings of Philip Yancey, Diane Jacobson, and Charles Spurgeon. Yancey states that the "point of the book is not suffering: Where is God when it hurts? The prologue dealt with that issue. The point is faith: Where is Job when it hurts?"[14] Jacobson rephrases this primary question as, "Does Job— does anyone—worship God for nothing, without wanting something in return? What makes the relationship of humans to God tick?"[15] Jacobson, who counts Job among the "'crushed theologians' . . . who cannot think their way to God but who are finally grasped by the cross"[16]—points out that Job and his friends share the same illusion that suffering is the result of sinning: "Job knows he is suffering, but he also knows that he is not 'evil' in a way that deserves such punishment. Therefore, because suffering is the result of punishment and the punishment should fit the crime, God is breaking the law. Like his friends, Job thinks that the world operates (or at least should operate) in an orderly manner."[17]

As Job loses his illusion and gains a new reality, he journeys from statements of faith to lamentations and from short declarations to agony-filled questions. His frustration-inspired, painfully honest truth-telling opens the way to greater intimacy with God. Jacobson explains,

> What he screams and laments for is relationship with God. He thinks perhaps that what he wants is some abstract revelation of truth and some answers as to why he is suffering. We share with Job his unquenchable desire to be given explanation and reasons for suffering. What Job gets is a relationship with God hidden within his remarkably odd encounter with God. . . . The final logic of Job is not the logic of justice but rather the logic of relationship. Knowing God, for Job, is deeply a matter of faith through suffering within the void. Chaos is taken up into the promise of God, and the only doorway is cloaked in darkness.[18]

In his study of Job, Spurgeon's conclusions concur: sorrow and weakness open the way to greater intimacy with God via a "fuller revelation of God."[19] Spurgeon explains that God "draws the curtain about the bed of his chosen sufferer and, at the same time he withdraws another curtain which aforetime concealed his glory."[20] Spurgeon biographer Peter Morden offers the following from Spurgeon's message on the book of Job:

> In a sermon entitled "Job Among The Ashes," he insisted that a believer's suffering could lead to a clearer sight of God. Prosperity was a "painted window" which shut out "the clear light of God." Only when the paint was removed did the window become "transparent," enabling God to be seen with a new clarity. This had been Job's experience: he had lost everything and this "paved the way" to his receiving a fuller revelation of God.[21]

Yancey also concurs regarding the outcome of Job's disillusionment, offering that "Paradoxically, the most perplexing, Job-like times may help 'fertilize' faith and nurture intimacy with God."[22]

FREUD, WEBER, AND HOMANS ON MOURNING AND DE-IDEALIZATION

More than these writers, however, our current understanding of spiritual pain has been shaped by a different era of both Christian and secular thinkers who exalted the very faculty earlier religious writers felt must be darkened to experience greater depths of the knowledge of God: the intellect.

Sigmund Freud, who is considered the founding father of psychoanalysis, developed theories that have influenced centuries of thought. Freud's concept of *mourning*—as the loss of a person, abstraction, or ideal[23]—and *de-idealization*[24] clearly overlap with disillusionment as defined in this book.

Whereas Freud seems to primarily address the mourning and de-idealization of individuals, Homans layers Weber's sociological thoughts over those of Freudian psychotherapy and offers an additional communal lens through which to process de-idealization. In fact, Homans claims that psychoanalysis is humanity's "creative response" to "a long, historical mourning process begun centuries ago, with roots in the origins of physical science in the seventeenth century and in the theology of the fourteenth."[25]

In other words, secularization—the steady shedding of religious meaning—replaced Judeo-Christian belief systems with psychoanalysis.

By explaining why religion was needed in the past, psychoanalysis rendered further need of religion superfluous. As summarized by Homans, "Freud and Jones accepted this metaphor of a war [between science and theology] . . . which was prominent in their day, and they conceived of the psychoanalytic movement as a kind of 'D-Day,' the final, decisive victory of the forces of good over those of evil."[26] For those aligned with Freud, the de-idealization, or loss, of Western religious "illusions" of a monotheistic God freed humanity to evolve into higher forms of thought.

Robert Merton, however, points out that theology was initially a generous benefactor, not a stingy detractor, of science,[27] and that the first scientists were most often men of deep faith who

> laud[ed] the faculty of reason. . . . Reason is praiseworthy because man, chosen of God, alone possesses it; it serves to differentiate him from the beasts of the field. . . . it possesses still another exemplary characteristic; it enables man more fully to glorify God by aiding him to appreciate His works. . . . Hence, it becomes imperative for them who would rationalize these doctrines to "prove" that *reason* and *faith*—two such highly exalted virtues of the Puritan—are not inconsistent.[28]

Surely few could foresee that this seventeenth-century theological celebration of reason would one day undermine the very belief systems that offered the celebration credibility! As Homans succinctly summarizes, "As they rationalized and disenchanted the biblical Christian world of spirit, the Puritan scientists turned to nature and matter. . . . [Later in] the hands of psychoanalysis, spirit becomes psyche and, still further, psyche becomes ego. The ego of psychoanalysis is simply the naturalization of the soul."[29]

Though uniquely applied to psychological human development, deidealization serves as a near synonym for disillusionment, for it involves both the loss of ideals and the interaction of mind and soul. However, disillusionment is not the loss of oneness with another human, but rather the journey to oneness with God. Spiritual disillusionment is not a crucible for self-consciousness but a crucible for God-consciousness. Obviously, self-consciousness and God-consciousness grow together in a human soul. But a fundamental definitional difference exists when one believes that there is a God to become conscious of and, further, that through God-consciousness, the God-follower emerges into a truer self. This view is in direct conflict with a more secular perspective that considers God-consciousness as the true illusion and, consequently, as a hindrance to the development of a healthy self.

Which is why Homans speaks of *mourning* and *meaning* as bridged by *individuation*. Homans explains that individuation is

> the fruit of mourning. Somehow, in a way that is not really understood, the experience of loss can stimulate the desire "to become who one is." That in turn can throw into motion a third process, what should be called "the creation of meaning." This action is at once a work of personal growth and a work of culture. In it, the self both appropriates from the past what has been lost and at the same time actually creates for itself in a fresh way these meanings.[30]

REITMAN, HARTT, VASSADY, AND BLUMENTHAL ON DESPAIR

Many scholars have written insightfully about *theological despair*. James S. Reitman, linking despair and disillusionment, states: "Despair [is] the ultimate logical outcome of profound disillusionment."[31] Theologian Julian Norris Hartt adds that despair can be understood in terms of illusions and actualities:

> Such a time is the occasion we have called despair, in which men reflect on the actualities of the human situation, and cower before a threatening world. We can no longer pretend that the threats are illusions, we can no longer deny that despair is well-grounded.[32]

Despair captures a fear of "discontinuity" of "being."[33] Discontinuity is when reason—defined by Hartt as "our will to domesticate the world, to tame its powers and harness its potencies"[34]—must bow to actualities like mortality. For example, we can build, and build beautifully, but in all our building we cannot give life nor can we prevent death.[35] All human strength will one day bow to the actuality of the grave. As Hartt states, "Revelation is something and Someone sweeping in over our well-mannered expectations. . . . God has the last word, and dams enough and strong enough cannot be erected against its shattering utterance."[36]

Hungarian theologian Béla Vassady associates disillusionment with the "sorrow of the world"—a despair that leads to death. Referring to despair as a philosophy, Vassady crafts a theology of hope to post–World War II Europeans. His theology of hope stands in contrast to the "human self-delusion" of "atheistic existentialism [in which the human person seeks to] rescue himself from his own despair."[37] With insight for then and now, Vassady asserts,

> Speaking in theological terms, the Christian refers to the fact
> that we cannot free ourselves "horizontally," i.e. by any amount
> of merely human endeavors. No human achievement, whether
> individual or collective, can ever bring us peace of mind. We
> must be lifted from above, from the vertical dimension. And it is
> Christ, who lifts us through his Word and Holy Spirit.[38]

For those suffering despair, hope is a vertical gift, not a horizontal achievement. Peace is found as we are "lifted from above."

Another offering from the ashes of World War II comes from Rabbi David R. Blumenthal. In a deeply moving contribution, Rabbi Blumenthal addresses theological despair by pressing readers to decide who bears responsibility for the Holocaust:

> Most religious folk, and most religious thinkers and clergy along
> with them, do not want to ask this question. They do not want
> to know that God is responsible for history, that is, for the bad
> parts.[39]

If you are religious, what do you think? Are you among the pious avoiders? Among those who say that God could not have been involved because God gave humankind a free will, an act which relieves God of all responsibility? Are you among those who believe that God is too good to be responsible? That God was absent? Or, are you among the heretical avoiders? Among those who deal with this question by denying God? You must take a stand, if God is integral to who you are.[40]

Blumenthal argues that, if unprocessed, theological despair leads to secularization, to heresy, and a "new form of self-hatred."[41] Both Vassady's hope in the vertical and Blumenthal's discussion on unprocessed despair correlate with the cycle of disillusionment.

SICKNESS UNTO DEATH, ANGST, AND THE ABSENCE THAT SANCTIFIES FROM KIERKEGAARD AND MERTON

Also related to disillusionment's loss of false ideas and gaining of reality is the Kierkegaardian concept of *Sickness unto Death*, or *Despair*. Writing under the name of Anti-Climacus, Kierkegaard asserts that through the very experience of loss, "there is also an essential advance made in the consciousness of the self."[42] Kierkegaardian despair[43] seems sourced less in the loss of illusions about God and more in the gaining of reality about self and, more specifically, in Kierkegaard's own personal search for the divine rest that only forgiveness can bring. Simon D. Podmore insightfully identifies the "dialectical polarities of forgiveness and despair" in Kierkegaard's writings that reflect his "need and desire to be delivered from despair and reconciled with forgiveness."[44]

Even closer, perhaps, to this book's definition of disillusionment is Kierkegaard's concept of existential *Angest* or *Anfægtelse*, which Podmore describes as a spiritual trial in which one becomes "conscious of the fact that one exists before God" and aware of the "'infinite qualitative difference' between self and God."[45] This gaining of reality—of the humanly insurmountable difference between the sinful self and a holy God—can lead to despair. Podmore explains that "if guilt over sin advances into depressive, fantastic, or pathological realms, then it risks giving birth to supplementary but no less harrowing forms of despair: namely, that which Kierkegaard himself had evidently labored under, despair over sins and despair of the forgiveness of sins."[46] Kierkegaard experienced disillusionment with his own self. When illusions about one's ability to follow God collide with the reality of human sinfulness, the soul—if not able or willing to receive the grace of forgiveness—can easily spiral toward theological despair.

Twentieth-century Trappist monk Thomas Merton also addressed the spiritual pain that sometimes accompanies disillusionment in his writing on *the two absences of God*, from which I will quote at length:

> God, Who is everywhere, never leaves us. Yet He seems sometimes to be present, sometimes absent. If we do not know Him well, we do not realize that He may be more present to us when He is absent than when He is present.

> There are two absences of God. One is an absence that condemns us, the other an absence that sanctifies us.

> In the absence that is condemnation, God "knows us not" because we have put some other god in His place, and refuse to be known by Him. In the absence that sanctifies, God empties the soul of every image that might become an idol and of every concern that might stand between our face and His Face.

> In the first absence, He is present, but His presence is denied by the presence of an idol. God is present to the enemy we have placed between ourselves and Him in mortal sin.

> In the second absence, He is present, and His presence is affirmed and adored by the absence of everything else. He is closer to us than we are to ourselves, although we do not see Him.[47]

Perhaps the pain of disillusionment's losses is reflected best in Merton's depiction of how "God empties the soul of every image that might become an idol . . . [and] stand between our face and His."

Surely the pain is well worth a clearer view of our Savior's face.

YANCEY ON DISAPPOINTMENT

Lastly in this brief summary of related terms, the contribution of Philip Yancey will be specifically considered. Though an esteemed editor and author, Yancey writes as an everyman, not as a scholar. His contributions are both thoughtful and substantial, and his writings have influenced the theology of millions, many of whom have yet to read the offerings of the above-mentioned scholars.

Via a walk through the Scriptures and his own personal experiences, Yancey addresses three disappointment-inducing questions: *Is God unfair? Is God silent?* and *Is God hidden?* From Yancey's perspective, our ability to be disappointed with God—our capacity to experience and verbalize disillusionment—is only possible because of the "risk" God took in creating us "free."[48]

God knew He would pay dearly when He chose to give us free will.

As Douglas John Hall has stated,

> God's problem is not that God *is not able* to do certain things.
> God's problem is that God loves! Love complicates the life
> of God as it complicates every life. Without love, [God could]
> behave towards the world in the way that . . . many other people
> seem to think desirable—punishing the evil-doers and rewarding
> the good (except that then . . . we might find a good deal more
> suffering in the world than we do now!). But, 'like as a father
> pitieth his children,' the biblical God is prevented from such

direct action because of a love which is ready to suffer with and for the beloved before it will give way to strict justice.[49]

We are free to love God. We are free to not love God.

And, in Yancey's words, "true, unbribed, freely offered faith [has] an intrinsic value to God that we can barely imagine."[50]

Through his writings, Yancey draws our attention to the unseen world. When disappointed, our choices affect invisible realms:

> Our choices matter, not just to us and our own destiny but, amazingly, to God himself and the universe he rules. . . . Our very existence announces to the powers in the universe that restoration is under way. Every act of faith by every one of the people of God is like the tolling of a bell, and a faith like Job's reverberates throughout the universe.[51]

Such an emphasis on freedom and the unseen world calls to mind the insightful dialogue between an elder demon and a younger demon in C. S. Lewis's *The Screwtape Letters*:

> The Enemy allows this disappointment to occur on the threshold of every human endeavor. . . . [He] takes this risk because He has a curious fantasy of making all these disgusting little human vermin into what He calls His "free" lovers and servants—"sons" is the word He uses. . . . Desiring their freedom, He therefore refuses to carry them, by their mere affections and habits, to any of the goals which He sets before them . . . remember, there lies our danger. If once they get through this initial dryness successfully, they become much less dependent on emotion and therefore much harder to tempt.[52]

In summary, many voices have shaped our understanding of spiritual pain. Sadly, we seem more formed today by trending podcasts than by profound thought.[53] Wisdom invites us to recall deeper voices that receive resonance from Eternity. Through history, great thinkers like Pseudo-Dionysius, John of the Cross, Thomas Merton, C. S. Lewis, and Philip Yancey agree: the purpose of the *darkness*, the *dark night*, the *absence*, and the *disappointment* is to purify and empower the soul to know a new dimension of intimacy with God.

Notes

CHAPTER 1: FACING THE STORM TOGETHER

1. Thanks for this, Dad. I miss you so much.

CHAPTER 2: NIGHT-FAITH

1. For a readable summary of a key study led by Jerome Siegel of UCLA, see Richard G. Stevens, "We Don't Need More Sleep. We Just Need More Darkness," *Washington Post*, October 27, 2015, https://www.washingtonpost.com/posteverything/wp /2015/10/27/we-dont-need-more-sleep-we-just-need-more-darkness/.

CHAPTER 3: THAT STARTLING "POP"

1. Though it had a slow start, *disillusionment* is far less of an uncommon word today. Of disillusionment, the *Oxford English Dictionary* states: "This word belongs in Frequency Band 5. Band 5 contains words which occur between 1 and 10 times per million words in typical modern English usage. These tend to be restricted to literate vocabulary associated with educated discourse." *Oxford English Dictionary Online*, s.v. "disillusionment (*noun*)," accessed July 26, 2022, https://www.oed .com/view/Entry/54538.

2. *Oxford English Dictionary Online*, s.v. "dis- (*prefix*)," accessed July 26, 2022, https://www.oed.com/view/Entry/53379.

3. Unlike *illusion*, *disillusion* is listed in neither the 1806 nor the 1828 edition of *Webster's Dictionary*. In 1913, *disillusion* was defined as "the act or process of freeing from an illusion." See *Webster's Revised Unabridged Dictionary*, s.v. "disillusion (*verb*)," accessed July 26, 2022, http://machaut.uchicago.edu/?resource=Webster %27s&word=disillusion&use1913=on. In 1980, *disillusion* was defined as "to disenchant or to free from illusion;" see the *New Webster Encyclopedic Dictionary of the English Language*, ed. Virginia S. Thatcher and Alexander McQueen (Chicago: Consolidated Book, 1980), s.v. "disillusion (*verb*)," 249. In 2014, *disillusion* was defined by *Merriam-Webster* as "the condition of being disenchanted," *Merriam-Webster*, s.v. "disillusion (*noun*)," accessed July 26, 2022, https://www.merriam -webster.com/dictionary/disillusion; and by the *Oxford English Dictionary* as "the

action of freeing or becoming freed from illusion; the condition of being freed from illusion; disenchantment," *Oxford English Dictionary Online*, s.v. "disillusion (*noun*)," accessed July 26, 2022, https://www.oed.com/view/Entry/54534.

4. *Oxford English Dictionary Online*, s.v. "illusion (*noun*)," accessed July 26, 2022, https://www.oed.com/view/Entry/91565.

5. *Oxford English Dictionary Online*, s.v. "-ment (*suffix*)," accessed July 26, 2022, https://www.oed.com/view/Entry/116535.

6. Or as a friend, Joe Zickafoose (d. 2008), succinctly summarized while I was teaching a small group on the subject, disillusionment is the "dissing of illusions."

7. Oswald Chambers, *Baffled to Fight Better: Job and the Problem of Suffering* (Grand Rapids, MI: Discovery House, 1990), 50–51, 85.

8. C. S. Lewis, *Prince Caspian: The Return to Narnia* (London: Geoffrey Bles, 1951; New York: HarperCollins, 2005), 151–52. Citations refer to the HarperCollins edition.

9. Please see appendix A for my responses to five objections to this statement excerpted from my dissertation on the subject.

10. Dan B. Allender and Tremper Longman III, *The Cry of the Soul: How Our Emotions Reveal Our Deepest Questions about God* (Colorado Springs: NavPress, 1994), 24. Speaking of the power of reality, happiness psychologist Dr. Gordon Livingston states that if we view the past as "a theater of experience, some good and some bad, [it] opens up the possibility of growth and change." As quoted by Diana Butler Bass, *A People's History of Christianity: The Other Side of the Story* (New York: HarperOne, 2010), loc. 38650, Kindle.

CHAPTER 4: WHAT'S IN A WORD, PART ONE

1. Even then, only once (in Isaiah 20:5) did any of these four translations agree on the use of the word *disillusion* as an accurate translation from the Hebrew. Please see appendix B for a table citing these appearances.

2. For those intrigued by the evolution of words, a brief etymology of disillusionment can be found in appendix C.

3. Gerald G. May, *The Dark Night of the Soul: A Psychiatrist Explores the Connection between Darkness and Spiritual Growth* (San Francisco: HarperSanFrancisco, 2005), 16, 201. May notes that in addition to being quoted in John of the Cross's *The Ascent of Mount Carmel*, Dionysius's well-known writings were also referenced two hundred years earlier by the unnamed author of *The Cloud of Unknowing* and the Augustinian monk Walter Hilton.

4. Pseudo-Dionysius, *Dionysius the Areopagite: On the Divine Names and the Mystical Theology*, trans. C. E. Rolt, repr. (London, 1920; Whitefish, MT: Kessinger, 1992), 194. Christian Classics Ethereal Library, https://www.ccel.org/ccel/john_cross /dark_night.viii.ix.html.

5. Evelyn Underhill, ed., *The Cloud of Unknowing: The Classic of Medieval Mysticism* (Mineola, NY: Dover Publications, 2003), loc. 576, Kindle.

6. John of the Cross, *Dark Night of the Soul*, rev. ed., trans. and ed. E. Allison Peers (New York: Image Books, 1959), chap. 9, para. 2, Christian Classics Ethereal Library, https://www.ccel.org/ccel/john_cross/dark_night.viii.ix.html.

7. Georg Wilhelm Friedrich Hegel, *Phenomenology of Spirit*, trans. Arnold V. Miller (Oxford: Clarendon Press, 1977), 455–57, as quoted in Daniel Berthold-Bond, "Lunar Musings? An Investigation of Hegel's and Kierkegaard's Portraits of Despair," *Religious Studies* 34, no. 1 (March 1998): 36. See article in entirety for an interesting comparison of Hegel's and Kierkegaard's concepts of despair.

8. Berthold-Bond, "Lunar Musings?" 41.

9. Søren Kierkegaard, *Fear and Trembling and The Sickness unto Death*, trans. Walter Lowrie (Princeton, NJ: Princeton University Press, 2013), 269.

10. Kierkegaard, *Sickness unto Death*, 277–78.

11. Kierkegaard, *Sickness unto Death*, 271–77, as quoted in Berthold-Bond, "Lunar Musings?"

12. Kierkegaard, *Sickness unto Death*, 266, as quoted in Berthold-Bond, "Lunar Musings?"

13. Charles H. Spurgeon, "A Question for a Questioner," sermon, Metropolitan Tabernacle, Newington, May 31, 1885, no. 1843.

14. Peter J. Morden, "C. H. Spurgeon and Suffering," *Evangelical Review of Theology* 35, no. 4 (October 1, 2011): 306–25.

15. Sigmund Freud, "Mourning and Melancholia," in *The Standard Edition of the Complete Psychological Works of Sigmund Freud*, ed. James Strachey, vol. 14 (London: Hogarth Press, 1957), 243.

16. Peter Homans, *The Ability to Mourn: Disillusionment and the Social Origins of Psychoanalysis* (Chicago: University of Chicago Press, 1989), 26.

17. As Peter Homans states, "The personal but also universal experience of object loss underlies [all] these" terms. Homans, *Ability to Mourn*, 24.

18. Of his own experience, Yancey writes, "Disappointment with God does not come only in dramatic circumstances. For me, it also edges unexpectedly into the mundaneness of everyday life. . . . I have found that petty disappointments tend to accumulate over time, undermining my faith with a lava flow of doubt. I start to wonder whether God cares about everyday details—about me. I am tempted to pray less often, having concluded in advance that it won't matter. Or will it? My emotions and my faith waver. Once those doubts seep in, I am even less prepared for times of major crisis." Yancey, *Disappointment with God*, 22–23.

19. Homans, 26, 244.

20. Homans, 25, 228–29.

21. C. S. Lewis, *A Grief Observed* (San Francisco: HarperSanFrancisco, 2001), 78.

22. Béla Vassady, "A Theology of Hope for the Philosophy of Despair," *Theology Today* 5, no. 2 (July 1, 1948): 159.

23. Julian Norris Hartt, "The Significance of Despair in Contemporary Theology," *Theology Today* 13, no. 1 (April 1, 1956): 47.

24. Homans, *Ability to Mourn*, 24.

25. Thomas Merton, *No Man Is an Island* (New York: Harcourt, 1983), 237.

26. Homans, *Ability to Mourn*, 24.

27. Homans, 26.

28. David R. Blumenthal, "Despair and Hope Late in Post-Shoah Life," originally

published in *Bridges: An Interdisciplinary Journal of Theology, Philosophy, History, and Science* 6, nos. 3/4 (1999), DavidBlumenthal.org, http://davidblumenthal.org/DespairHope.html.

29. Blumenthal, "Despair and Hope."

30. May, *Dark Night*, 4–5.

31. Jerome T. Walsh, "Despair as a Theological Virtue in the Spirituality of Ecclesiastes," *Biblical Theology Bulletin* 12, no. 2 (April 1982): 47.

32. James S. Reitman, "God's 'Eye' for the *Imago Dei*: Wise Advocacy amid Disillusionment in Job and Ecclesiastes," *Trinity Journal* 31, no. 1 (March 1, 2010): 115–16.

33. Philip Yancey, *Disappointment with God: Three Questions No One Asks Aloud* (Grand Rapids, MI: Zondervan, 1988), 9.

34. Yancey, 37.

35. Gene Edward Veith Jr., *Loving God with All Your Mind: Thinking as a Christian in the Postmodern World*, rev. ed. (Wheaton, IL: Crossway Books, 2003), 51.

36. Berthold-Bond, "Lunar Musings?" 36.

37. Elie Kaplan Spitz with Erica Shapiro Taylor, *Healing from Despair: Choosing Wholeness in a Broken World* (Woodstock, VT: Jewish Lights, 2008), 35.

38. John H. Coe, "Musings on the Dark Night of the Soul: Insights from St. John of the Cross on a Developmental Spirituality," *Journal of Psychology and Theology* 28, no. 4 (2000): 293.

39. Simon D. Podmore, "Lazarus and the Sickness unto Death: An Allegory of Despair," *Religion and the Arts* 15, no. 4 (January 1, 2011): 487.

CHAPTER 5: WHAT'S IN A WORD, PART TWO

1. *Oxford English Dictionary Online*, s.v. "cynic (*noun*)," accessed July 26, 2022, https://www.oed.com/view/Entry/46638.

2. Oswald Chambers, "The Discipline of Disillusionment," *My Utmost for His Highest* (Uhrichsville, OH: Barbour, 1991), July 30th.

3. For an interesting history of skepticism, see Katja Vogt, "Ancient Skepticism," *Stanford Encyclopedia of Philosophy* (summer 2021 edition), ed. Edward N. Zalta, Stanford University, article published February 24, 2010, last revised July 20, 2018, https://plato.stanford.edu/archives/sum2021/entries/skepticism-ancient/.

4. *Oxford English Dictionary Online*, s.v. "sceptic | skeptic (*noun*)," accessed July 26, 2022, https://www.oed.com/view/Entry/172249.

5. Also known as *Home of the Gentry* and *A House of Gentlefolk*. In 1894 it was translated into English by Constance Clara Garnett (1861–1946).

6. Ivan Sergeevich Turgenev, *A Nest of Gentry*, in *The Essential Turgenev*, ed. Elizabeth Cheresh Allen (Evanston, IL: Northwestern University Press, 1994), 397–98.

7. *Merriam-Webster*, s.v. "skepticism (*noun*)," accessed July 25, 2022, https://www.merriam-webster.com/dictionary/skepticism.

8. *APA Dictionary of Psychology*, s.v. "despair (*noun*)," accessed July 25, 2022, https://dictionary.apa.org/despair.

9. For a brief consideration of despair, disillusionment, and suicide, please see Objection Four in appendix A.

10. Abraham J. Twerski, foreword to Elie Kaplan Spitz with Erica Shapiro Taylor, *Healing from Despair: Choosing Wholeness in a Broken World* (Woodstock, VT: Jewish Lights, 2008), xv.

CHAPTER 6: A RELATIONAL CYCLE

1. *Oxford English Dictionary Online*, s.v. "joy (*noun*)," accessed July 26, 2022, https://www.oed.com/view/Entry/101795.
2. *Merriam-Webster*, s.v. "anticipation (*noun*)," accessed July 26, 2022, https://www.merriam-webster.com/dictionary/anticipation.
3. Space sadly does not permit the exploration of correlations between joyful anticipation in particular (and the illustration in general) with Teresa of Ávila's first three mansions and Bernard of Clairvaux's first two degrees of love. See Teresa of Ávila, *Interior Castle*, trans. E. Allison Peers (Radford, VA: Wilder Publications, 2008); "Bernard Clairvaux on Love," Christian History Institute, accessed July 26, 2022, https://christianhistoryinstitute.org/study/module/bernard.
4. See Philippians 3:10 and 1 Peter 4:13.

CHAPTER 7: BETWEEN ILLUSION AND REALITY

1. *Oxford English Dictionary Online*, s.v. "no man's land (*noun*)," accessed July 28, 2022, https://www.oed.com/view/Entry/256795.
2. C. S. Lewis, *A Grief Observed* (San Francisco: HarperSanFrancisco, 2001), 78.
3. From a psychological perspective, Peter Homans explains, "Since history rarely optimally facilitates psychological development, such mergers are eventually challenged by interpersonal, social, and historical circumstances. As a result, the idealizations lose their firmness and may even crumble, leading to a weakened sense of self, a sense of betrayal, a conviction that an important value has been lost, moments of rage at the object (subsequently perceived as having failed the self in some way or other), and a consequent general sense of inner disorganization and paralysis." Peter Homans, *The Ability to Mourn: Disillusionment and the Social Origins of Psychoanalysis* (Chicago: University of Chicago Press, 1989), 24.
4. Gerald G. May, *The Dark Night of the Soul: A Psychiatrist Explores the Connection between Darkness and Spiritual Growth* (San Francisco: HarperSanFrancisco, 2005), 71. May explains why this process can be so agonizing: "We cling to things, people, beliefs, and behaviors not because we love them, but because we are terrified of losing them. The classical spiritual term for this compulsive condition is attachment. . . . All major spiritual traditions have long understood that attachment binds the energy of the human spirit to something other than love. Each of us has countless attachments. We are attached to our daily routines, our environments, our relationships, and of course our possessions. We are also attached to our religious beliefs and to our images of ourselves, others, and God." May, *Dark Night*, 60.
5. Søren Kierkegaard, *Fear and Trembling and The Sickness unto Death*, trans. Walter Lowrie (Princeton, NJ: Princeton University Press, 2013), 310.
6. John H. Coe, "Musings on the Dark Night of the Soul: Insights from St. John of

the Cross on a Developmental Spirituality," *Journal of Psychology and Theology* 28, no. 4 (2000): 304.

7. Contrasting Kierkegaard's movement away from reason and Hegel's movement toward reason (i.e., philosophical thought) to "cure" religious despair, philosophy professor Daniel Berthold-Bond notes that both "therapeutic leaps entail an act of sacrifice or renunciation or surrender" of the self, the will, and "I," which is where authentic faith, in Hegel's words, "'first finds its turning point.'" Daniel Berthold-Bond, "Lunar Musings? An Investigation of Hegel's and Kierkegaard's Portraits of Despair," *Religious Studies* 34, no. 1 (March 1998), 51.

CHAPTER 8: THE UPWARD PULL OF LOVE

1. Peter Homans, *The Ability to Mourn: Disillusionment and the Social Origins of Psychoanalysis* (Chicago: University of Chicago Press, 1989), 24.

2. Gerald G. May, *The Dark Night of the Soul: A Psychiatrist Explores the Connection between Darkness and Spiritual Growth* (San Francisco: HarperSanFrancisco, 2005), 67.

3. May, 47.

4. John H. Coe, "Musings on the Dark Night of the Soul: Insights from St. John of the Cross on a Developmental Spirituality," *Journal of Psychology and Theology* 28, no. 4 (2000): 295.

5. C. S. Lewis, *The World's Last Night, and Other Essays* (New York: Harcourt Brace, 1952; repr., San Francisco: HarperOne, 2017), 25–26.

CHAPTER 9: A CHOICE IN THE DARK

1. John H. Coe, "Musings on the Dark Night of the Soul: Insights from St. John of the Cross on a Developmental Spirituality," *Journal of Psychology and Theology* 28, no. 4 (2000): 301–2.

2. As Coe beautifully states, "The Christian life is more about Christ and less about our efforts. It is about what He has done, and about our life 'in Christ,' and how to open our hearts to this New Covenant life dependent upon the Spirit. This is an obedience of abiding in the Vine and opening to the Life of God living within. . . . As I grow [in the Christian] faith, I find that I am invited by the Spirit to learn to give up on the project of moralism, of trying to fix myself by my spiritual efforts. Rather, I want to open more deeply to Christ's work on the cross, and the Work of the Spirit in my deep for my daily bread." John H. Coe, "Resisting the Temptation of Moral Formation: Opening to Spiritual Formation in the Cross and the Spirit," *Journal of Spiritual Formation and Soul Care* 1, no. 1 (March 1, 2008): 57.

3. Gerald G. May, *The Dark Night of the Soul: A Psychiatrist Explores the Connection between Darkness and Spiritual Growth* (San Francisco: HarperSanFrancisco, 2005), 133.

4. Béla Vassady, "A Theology of Hope for the Philosophy of Despair," *Theology Today* 5, no. 2 (July 1, 1948): 162.

5. Anthony Reading distinguishes between faith and hope as follows: "Faith, a variant of hope, is based on belief rather than knowledge. Like hope, it involves positive

expectations about the future and generates behavior designed to help make its expectations come true. But the future-oriented behaviors that faith generates, such as prayer and ritual, require the intervention of a deity to achieve their desired outcome, in addition to the individual's own efforts. . . . While there is a certain logic to hope, albeit one that may often be apparent only to the beholder, faith does not require the same type of rationality to sustain it." Anthony Reading, *Hope and Despair: How Perceptions of the Future Shape Human Behavior* (Baltimore, MD: Johns Hopkins University Press, 2004), 8.

6. *Oxford English Dictionary Online*, s.v. "commitment (*noun*)," accessed July 29, 2022, https://www.oed.com/view/Entry/37161.

7. A poignant addition to this thought comes from Gregory of Nyssa in *Life of Moses*, 2.251–252, who said, "Moses, who eagerly seeks to behold God, is now taught how he can behold him: to follow God wherever he might lead is to behold God." Everett Ferguson, ed., *Inheriting Wisdom: Readings for Today from Ancient Christian Writers* (Peabody, MA: Hendrickson, 2004), 217.

8. May, speaking about the writings of John of the Cross, describes this process as follows: "In spiritual matters it is precisely when we *do* think we know where to go that we are most likely to stumble. Thus, John says, God darkens our awareness *in order to keep us safe*. When we cannot chart our own course, we become vulnerable to God's protection, and the darkness becomes a 'guiding night,' a 'night more kindly than the dawn.'" May, *Dark Night*, 72.

9. David R. Blumenthal, "Despair and Hope Late in Post-Shoah Life," originally published in *Bridges: An Interdisciplinary Journal of Theology, Philosophy, History, and Science* 6, nos. 3/4 (1999), 121, 122, 127, DavidBlumenthal.org, http://davidblumenthal.org/DespairHope.html.

10. Blumenthal, "Despair and Hope."

11. For any who may wonder, this baby did become a forever Chole.

12. Hebrews 11:39.

13. C. S. Lewis, *The Screwtape Letters: With Screwtape Proposes a Toast*, rev. ed. (New York: Collier Books, 1982), 39.

CHAPTER 10: A SPIRITUAL EXFOLIATE

1. John H. Coe, "Musings on the Dark Night of the Soul: Insights from St. John of the Cross on a Developmental Spirituality," *Journal of Psychology and Theology* 28, no. 4 (2000): 306.

2. Anthony Reading, *Hope and Despair: How Perceptions of the Future Shape Human Behavior* (Baltimore, MD: Johns Hopkins University Press, 2004), 17.

3. John H. Coe, "Resisting the Temptation of Moral Formation: Opening to Spiritual Formation in the Cross and the Spirit," *Journal of Spiritual Formation and Soul Care* 1, no. 1 (March 1, 2008): 61.

4. Philip Yancey, *Disappointment with God: Three Questions No One Asks Aloud* (Grand Rapids, MI: Zondervan, 1988), 66.

5. John H. Coe and Todd W. Hall, *Psychology in the Spirit: Contours of a Transformational Psychology* (Downers Grove, IL: IVP Academic, 2010), 288.

6. Shults and Sandage note, "Formed for the sake of self-protection, our egoistic love is not powerful enough either to bring us into right relations with others or to keep them from crushing or abandoning us." F. LeRon Shults and Steven J. Sandage, *Transforming Spirituality: Integrating Theology and Psychology* (Grand Rapids, MI: Baker Academic, 2006), 117.

7. As Rowan Williams notes, "In suffering, the believer's self-protection and isolation are broken." Rowan Williams, *The Wound of Knowledge: Christian Spirituality from the New Testament to St. John of the Cross*, 2nd rev. ed. (Cambridge, MA: Cowley Publications, 1991), 21.

CHAPTER 11: YELLOW JACKETS

1. Leonard Sweet, *The Well-Played Life: Why Pleasing God Doesn't Have to Be Such Hard Work* (Carol Stream, IL: Tyndale Momentum, 2014), 102.

2. Alicia Britt Chole, *40 Days of Decrease: A Different Kind of Hunger, a Different Kind of Fast* (Nashville: W Publishing Group, an imprint of Thomas Nelson, 2015), 22.

3. David R. Blumenthal, "Despair and Hope Late in Post-Shoah Life," originally published in *Bridges: An Interdisciplinary Journal of Theology, Philosophy, History, and Science* 6, nos. 3/4 (1999), DavidBlumenthal.org, http://davidblumenthal.org/DespairHope.html.

4. John of the Cross, *The Dark Night of the Soul*, in *Devotional Classics: Selected Readings for Individuals and Groups*, ed. Richard J. Foster and James Bryan Smith (San Francisco: HarperSanFrancisco, 1993), 33–34.

5. And yes, I agree. I hope Keona will write a book someday too.

CHAPTER 12: WHAT GOD WANTS

1. Oswald Chambers, *Baffled to Fight Better: Job and the Problem of Suffering* (Grand Rapids, MI: Discovery House, 1990), 14.

2. Chambers, 27.

CHAPTER 13: SOMETHING OLD

1. Appendix D includes brief summaries of brilliant thoughts on the books of Ecclesiastes and Job from Reitman, Walsh, Podmore, Yancey, Jacobson, and Spurgeon. Additionally, I highly recommend the out-of-print (which is perplexing) *Baffled to Fight Better: Job and the Problem of Suffering* by Oswald Chambers.

2. "As the Deer Panteth for the Water—written in 1984," *thescottspot* (blog), November 25, 2016, https://thescottspot.wordpress.com/2016/11/25/as-the-deer-panteth-for-the-water-written-in-1984/.

3. Martin J. Nystrom, "As the Deer," Universal Music/Brentwood-Benson Publishing, 1984.

4. "The great deep above stretches out its hand to the great deep below, and in voice of thunder their old relationship is recognised." Charles H. Spurgeon, "Deep Calleth unto Deep," sermon, Metropolitan Tabernacle, Newington, April 11, 1869, no. 865, The Spurgeon Center for Biblical Preaching at Midwestern

Seminary, https://www.spurgeon.org/resource-library/sermons/deep-calleth-unto
-deep/#flipbook/.

5. "This image was furnished by the windings and rapids of the Jordan." Anthony
Stocker Aglen, "Psalms," in *A Bible Commentary for English Readers*, ed. Charles
John Ellicott (London: Cassell, 1905), Ellicott's Commentary for English Readers,
Psalm 42, Bible Hub, https://biblehub.com/commentaries/ellicott/psalms/42.htm.

6. Alexander Francis Kirkpatrick, *Psalms: Books II & III*, Cambridge Bible for Schools
and Colleges, ed. J. J. S. Perowne (Cambridge: Cambridge University Press, 1904),
Psalm 42, Bible Hub, https://biblehub.com/commentaries/cambridge/psalms
/42.htm.

CHAPTER 16: GROWING PAINS

1. Whereas Part One was shaped mostly by research and citations, Parts Two, Three,
and Four will be shaped mostly by story and illustrations.

2. Chandler Moore, Chris Brown, Naomi Rain, and Steven Furtick, "Jireh," track 2
on *Old Church Basement*, Elevation Worship/Maverick City Music, released as a
single March 26, 2021.

3. Oswald Chambers, *Baffled to Fight Better: Job and the Problem of Suffering* (Grand
Rapids, MI: Discovery House, 1990), 38.

CHAPTER 17: COOKIES AND CANDOR

1. Consider Philippians 3:10; Colossians 1:24; 1 Peter 4:12-13.

2. Oswald Chambers, *Baffled to Fight Better: Job and the Problem of Suffering* (Grand
Rapids, MI: Discovery House, 1990), 26.

CHAPTER 18: WHAT DOTS ARE NOT

1. *Oxford English Dictionary Online* defines *effendi* as "a Turkish title of respect, chiefly
applied to government officials and members of the learned professions." *Oxford
Dictionary Online*, s.v. "effendi (*noun*)," accessed August 1, 2022, https://www.oed
.com/view/Entry/59711.

2. Oswald Chambers, *Leagues of Light: Diary of Oswald Chambers 1915–1917*
(Louisville, KY: Operation Appreciation Ministries, 1984), 85.

CHAPTER 21: IN THE MOURNING

1. The bulk of this chapter first appeared in a book that is now out of print. Alicia
Britt Chole, *Sitting in God's Sunshine, Resting in His Love* (Nashville: JCountryman,
2005), 150–54.

CHAPTER 23: A LIFELINE

1. Dickinson to Mrs. Henry Hills, ca. 1884, in Richard B. Sewall, *The Life of Emily
Dickinson*, 2 vols. (Cambridge, MA: Harvard University Press, 1994), 2:461.

2. *Oxford English Dictionary Online*, s.v. "activate (*verb*)," accessed August 2, 2022,
https://www.oed.com/view/Entry/1952.

3. Thanks to Rosie O'neal for this fabulous phrase.

CHAPTER 24: THE UNGLAMOROUS GIFT

1. Kathleen Norris, *The Cloister Walk* (New York: Riverhead Books, 1996), 363.
2. See John D. Woodbridge, ed., *Ambassadors for Christ: Distinguished Representatives of the Message throughout the World* (Chicago: Moody, 1994), 20–29.
3. Carey to Andrew Fuller, 1812, in Kellsye M. Finnie, *William Carey: By Trade a Cobbler* (Eastbourne, England: Kingsway, 1986), 129. See also E. Michael Rusten and Sharon O. Rusten, *The One Year Book of Christian History* (Wheaton, IL: Tyndale, 2003).
4. William Carey, as quoted in Woodbridge, *Ambassadors for Christ*, 29.
5. *Oxford English Dictionary Online*, s.v. "plod (*verb*)," accessed August 2, 2022, https://www.oed.com/view/Entry/145877.
6. Erica R. Hendry, "7 Epic Fails Brought to You by the Genius Mind of Thomas Edison," *Smithsonian*, November 20, 2013, https://www.smithsonianmag.com/innovation/7-epic-fails-brought-to-you-by-the-genius-mind-of-thomas-edison-180947786/.
7. Nelson Mandela, *Long Walk to Freedom: The Autobiography of Nelson Mandela* (New York: Little, Brown, 1995), 566.

CHAPTER 26: SPIRITUAL FRUSTRATION

1. Lexico, s.v. "frustration (*noun*)," accessed August 2, 2022, https://www.lexico.com/en/definition/frustration.
2. *Oxford English Dictionary Online*, s.v. "frustrate (*verb*)," accessed August 2, 2022, https://www.oed.com/view/Entry/75139.
3. *Oxford English Dictionary Online*, s.v. "frustration (*noun*)," accessed August 2, 2022, https://www.oed.com/view/Entry/75142.
4. Vocabulary.com, s.v. "frustrating (*adjective*)," accessed August 2, 2022, https://www.vocabulary.com/dictionary/frustrating.
5. Thanks to Jennifer Day for this fun phrase.

CHAPTER 27: SOMETHING OLD

1. Alicia Britt Chole, "Enthroning Truth," talk given as part of the DVD set *Choices: To Be or Not to Be a Woman of God* (Rogersville, MO: onewholeworld, 2003).
2. Oswald Chambers, *Leagues of Light: Diary of Oswald Chambers 1915–1917* (Louisville, KY: Operation Appreciation Ministries, 1984), 86.
3. One of my mentors, Gail MacDonald, helped me greatly in this regard. She reminded me that the amygdala's job is to record emotionally painful experiences and then alert me—through fear and anxiety—when a situation even remotely resembled the initial trauma. She said something like, "Remember, Alicia, these emotions indicate that your amygdala is just doing its job. BUT it's responding to your past, not predicting your future."

CHAPTER 28: SOMETHING NEW

1. Alicia Britt Chole, *40 Days of Decrease: A Different Kind of Hunger, a Different Kind of Fast* (Nashville: W Publishing Group, an imprint of Thomas Nelson, 2015), 154.
2. Chole, 155.

CHAPTER 29: CHASING HORSES

1. Oswald Chambers, *Baffled to Fight Better: Job and the Problem of Suffering* (Grand Rapids, MI: Discovery House, 1990), 131–32.
2. Robert Robinson, "Come Thou Fount," 1757.
3. "File: Robert Robinson.jpg," Wikimedia Commons, last updated October 26, 2020, https://commons.wikimedia.org/wiki/File:Robert_Robinson.jpg. Anonymous, cropped image in Edwin M. Long, *Illustrated History of Hymns and Their Authors* (1875), 344.
4. Jerry B. Jenkins, *Hymns for Personal Devotions* (Chicago: Moody, 1989), 78.
5. Kenneth W. Osbeck, *101 Hymn Stories: The Inspiring True Stories behind 101 Favorite Hymns* (Grand Rapids, MI: Kregel, 2012), 52.
6. If you have done the same, you know the feeling. I can only describe it as *cold*. And I can only guess that insanity is a short walk down the street.

CHAPTER 30: HEART MATTERS

1. Note that Jesus takes up part of this jeremiad in Matthew 15:8, when He says, "These people honor me with their lips, but their hearts are far from me."
2. I.e., *grow* (72), *growers* (1), *growing* (13), *grown* (21), *grows* (23), and *growth* (3). Interestingly, 110 of the 133 occurrences are found in the Old Testament, with the highest concentrations in the following books: Isaiah (19), Psalms (13), and Job (10). *NIV Hebrew-Greek Key Word Study Bible* (Chattanooga, TN: AMG Publishers, 1996).
3. The greatest concentrations can be found in Matthew (6) and Colossians (4).
4. See Matthew 24:12 (love growing cold); 1 Corinthians 3:6-7, 2 Corinthians 10:15, and 2 Thessalonians 1:3 (faith); Ephesians 4:15-16 and Colossians 2:19 (the body of Christ growing); Colossians 1:6 (the gospel is growing); Colossians 1:10 (growing in knowledge); 1 Peter 2:2 (growing up in salvation); 2 Peter 3:18 (growing in grace).

CHAPTER 31: THAT SAME OLD SPOT

1. D. W. Lambert, *Oswald Chambers: An Unbribed Soul* (1983; repr., Fort Washington, PA: Christian Literature Crusade, 1989), 66.
2. "He's Changing Me," author and date unknown.

CHAPTER 32: GAINING GROUND

1. Occurring only between .01 to .1 times per million words uttered today. See *Oxford English Dictionary Online*, s.v. "besetting (*adjective*)," accessed August 4, 2022, https://www.oed.com/view/Entry/18055.
2. Robert Southey, *Joan of Arc*, rev. ed. (1796; London: Longman, Orme, Brown, 1841), 2.69.
3. *Oxford English Dictionary Online*, s.v. "beset (*verb*)," accessed August 4, 2022, https://www.oed.com/view/Entry/18051.
4. *Oxford English Dictionary Online*, s.v. "victory (*noun*)," accessed August 4, 2022, https://www.oed.com/view/Entry/223235.

CHAPTER 33: NEVER WASTED

1. Dr. Tom Rundell, ca. 2012.

CHAPTER 34: FILTERING "FAILURES"

1. *Merriam-Webster*, s.v. "failure (*noun*)," accessed August 4, 2022, https://www.merriam-webster.com/dictionary/failure.
2. Though often attributed to Winston Churchill, the original source of this quote is unknown.

CHAPTER 35: PICKLE SOUP

1. *Encyclopedia Britannica*, s.v. "Incarnation," August 4, 2022, https://www.britannica.com/topic/Incarnation-Jesus-Christ.
2. See Alicia Britt Chole, *Anonymous: Jesus' Hidden Years . . . and Yours* (Franklin, TN: Integrity, 2006), 80.

CHAPTER 36: THE COMMON THREAD

1. Lewis B. Smedes, *Shame and Grace: Healing the Shame We Don't Deserve* (San Francisco: HarperSanFrancisco, 1993), 109.
2. Smedes, 116.
3. Smedes, 117–18.
4. Precept Austin, "Grace—Charis (Greek Word Study)," updated August 11, 2020, italics added, https://www.preceptaustin.org/grace_charis.
5. *Oxford English Dictionary Online*, s.v. "performance (*noun*)," accessed August 4, 2022, https://www.oed.com/view/Entry/140783.
6. *Oxford English Dictionary Online*, s.v. "pilgrimage (*noun*)," accessed August 4, 2022, https://www.oed.com/view/Entry/143868.

CHAPTER 38: (NOT SO) WELL WITH MY SOUL

1. This summary is drawn from the following sources: Rachael Phillips, *Well with My Soul: Four Dramatic Stories of Great Hymn Writers* (Uhrichsville, OH: Barbour, 2003); Bertha Spafford Vester, *Our Jerusalem: An American Family in the Holy City, 1881–1949* (LaVergne, TN: Ramsay Press, 2007); Wikipedia, s.v. "Horatio Spafford," last modified May 4, 2022, https://en.wikipedia.org/wiki/Horatio_Spafford; The Spafford Children's Center, "History," accessed August 4, 2022, https://spaffordcenter.org/about-us/history/.
2. Phillips, *Well with My Soul*, 31.
3. Some sources mention two sons, both named Horatio, who died of scarlet fever between the ages of three and four. I have tried to remain true to the family's official account, which only mentions one son named Horatio. After Horatio's death, the Spaffords were blessed with another daughter, whom they named Grace.
4. Phillips, *Well with My Soul*, 44.
5. Oswald Chambers, *Baffled to Fight Better: Job and the Problem of Suffering* (Grand Rapids, MI: Discovery House, 1990), 23.
6. Spafford Vester, *Our Jerusalem*, 54.

7. Phillips, *Well with My Soul*, 44.
8. What they planted still endures today as the Spafford Children's Center in Jerusalem. For more information, visit the Spafford Children's Center online, https://spaffordcenter.org/.
9. Spafford Vester, *Our Jerusalem*, 55.

CHAPTER 40: SUNDAY SCHOOLED

1. Peter Scholtes, "They'll Know We Are Christians by Our Love," 1966, F.E.L. Publications, assigned to the Lorenz Corp., 1991.

CHAPTER 44: TABLE STRETCHES

1. Mental flexibility "is about personal adaptability and our willingness to shift our thought patterns to respond to given situations in less regimented ways. . . . Our mind is like a muscle, the more ways that we stretch it, the more flexible it becomes. With practice and awareness, we can begin to develop a more agile mind which helps us to live more resilient, creative and fulfilled lives." "Mental Flexibility," Prospect Medical, accessed August 5, 2022, https://www.prospectmedical.com/resources/wellness-center/mental-flexibility.

CHAPTER 45: TO HAVE, OR NOT TO HAVE, A COW

1. Scott and Crystal Martin. Shared with permission.
2. Edwin H. Friedman, *Generation to Generation: Family Process in Church and Synagogue* (New York: Guilford, 2011), 27.

CHAPTER 46: A MUSCULAR MERCY

1. For more on this desert retreat, see chapter 16, and visit the Evangelical Sisterhood of Mary USA's Prayer Garden Tour online, https://www.canaaninthedesert.com/.
2. See Matthew 15:7-9 and Matthew 23.

CHAPTER 47: WHAT WAS, WAS

1. *Oxford English Dictionary Online*, s.v. "revisionism (*noun*)," accessed August 6, 2022, https://www.oed.com/view/Entry/164895.
2. Kristen Utter, letter to author, February 2, 2022. Used with permission. She has written a book about her experience entitled *Shatterproof: What Held Me Together When My World Fell Apart* (Magnolia, TX: Lucid Books, 2022).

CHAPTER 48: THE "SHOW ME" STATE

1. Wikipedia, s.v. "It takes two to tango," last updated June 5, 2022, https://en.wikipedia.org/wiki/It_takes_two_to_tango.

CHAPTER 49: FROM ABOVE

1. Augustine, *Expositions on the Book of Psalms*, vol. 1 (Oxford, 1847), Psalm 31, sermon 3, verse 15.
2. *Oxford English Dictionary Online*, s.v. "mercenary (*adjective*)," accessed August 6, 2022, https://www.oed.com/view/Entry/116635.

CHAPTER 52: CONCLUSION

1. Gerald G. May, *The Dark Night of the Soul: A Psychiatrist Explores the Connection between Darkness and Spiritual Growth* (San Francisco: HarperSanFrancisco, 2005), 132.

2. Alicia Britt Chole, *Finding an Unseen God: Reflections of a Former Atheist* (Bloomington, MN: Bethany House, 2008), 111.

3. Oswald Chambers, *Baffled to Fight Better: Job and the Problem of Suffering* (Grand Rapids, MI: Discovery House, 1990), 130.

APPENDIX A: OBJECTIONS

1. Deanna A. Thompson, *Crossing the Divide: Luther, Feminism, and the Cross* (Minneapolis, MN: Fortress, 2004), ix.

2. Thompson, 100.

3. Philip Yancey, *Disappointment with God: Three Questions No One Asks Aloud* (Grand Rapids, MI: Zondervan, 1988), 24.

4. Yancey, 26.

5. Julian Norris Hartt, "The Significance of Despair in Contemporary Theology," *Theology Today* 13, no. 1 (April 1, 1956): 61.

6. See 1 Thessalonians 1:4-6; James 1:2-4, 12; 1 Peter 1:6-7; 4:12-14.

7. Matthew 27:46.

8. Luke 23:46.

9. Peter L. Steinke, *How Your Church Family Works: Understanding Congregations as Emotional Systems* (Herndon, VA: Alban Institute, 2006), xiv.

10. Coe offers the following on distinguishing between a dark night and depression: "From an objective standpoint, the dark night is a movement of the Spirit on behalf of the believer, whereas clinical depression can have a more historical or biological etiology. From a subjective viewpoint, depression may involve no particular object or focus other than a diffused sense of loss of pleasure, a difficulty in sleep, a generally depressed mood, and overall energy loss. The dark night, on the contrary, has a more refined focus, namely, upon one's relationship with God, which is particularly brought into view in the practice of the spiritual disciplines (prayer, reading the Bible, fellowship, hearing preaching, worship). If there is a generally depressed mood while in a dark night, it can be brought into sharper focus to distinguish between feelings that emerge in relation to the spiritual life alone and those that persist in general. Interestingly, a believer in a dark night, instead of feeling depressed, may feel quite energized in life's activities in general and, as a result, repress the religious dimension in light of the fact that this is the objective focus of the internal turmoil." John H. Coe, "Musings on the Dark Night of the Soul: Insights from St. John of the Cross on a Developmental Spirituality," *Journal of Psychology and Theology* 28, no. 4 (2000): 306–7.

11. Anthony Reading, *Hope and Despair: How Perceptions of the Future Shape Human Behavior* (Baltimore, MD: Johns Hopkins University Press, 2004), x.

12. Reading, 151.

13. Reading, 151.
14. Reading, 153.
15. Reading, 150.
16. For an intriguing diagram of the relationship between hope and depression, see Reading, 19.
17. Reading, 155.
18. Elie Kaplan Spitz with Erica Shapiro Taylor, *Healing from Despair: Choosing Wholeness in a Broken World* (Woodstock, VT: Jewish Lights, 2008), 43.
19. Søren Kierkegaard, *Fear and Trembling and The Sickness unto Death*, trans. Walter Lowrie (Princeton, NJ: Princeton University Press, 2013), 358.
20. Abraham J. Twerski, foreword to Spitz, *Healing from Despair*, xiii.
21. Spitz, 22–24.
22. Spitz, 10.
23. Spitz, 3.
24. Spitz, 40.
25. Gene Edward Veith Jr., *Loving God with All Your Mind: Thinking as a Christian in the Postmodern World*, rev. ed. (Wheaton, IL: Crossway Books, 2003), 49.
26. Veith, 50.
27. Veith, 51.
28. Veith, 49.
29. *Merriam-Webster*, s.v. "objective (*adjective*)," accessed August 6, 2022, https://www.merriam-webster.com/dictionary/objective.
30. From a psychiatric perspective, Anthony Reading adds that the "mental models we construct can never fully apprehend reality, because our systems of knowledge and understanding are all built on initial beliefs that cannot themselves be proven. We have to take something for granted before we can understand something else, to start with an initial point of reference that we accept implicitly before we can institute logical operations." Reading, *Hope and Despair*, 32.
31. Reading, 150.
32. Spitz, *Healing from Despair*, 14.
33. Yancey, *Disappointment with God*, 204.
34. Reading, *Hope and Despair*, x.
35. C. S. Lewis, *The Screwtape Letters: With Screwtape Proposes a Toast*, rev. ed. (New York: Collier Books, 1982), 141.
36. C. H. Spurgeon, *The Autobiography of Charles H. Spurgeon: Compiled from His Diary, Letters, and Records by His Wife and His Private Secretary*, vol. 2 (Chicago: Fleming H. Revell, 1899), 220.
37. Peter J. Morden, "C. H. Spurgeon and Suffering," *Evangelical Review of Theology* 35, no. 4 (October 1, 2011): 309.
38. Charles H. Spurgeon, "A Question for a Questioner," sermon, Metropolitan Tabernacle, Newington, May 31, 1885, no. 1843, https://ccel.org/ccel/spurgeon/sermons31/sermons31.iv_1.html.

APPENDIX B: OCCURRENCES OF *DISILLUSION* IN ENGLISH TRANSLATIONS OF THE BIBLE

1. Two additional English translations make use of *disillusion/disillusioned/disillusionment,* but as a chapter title (see Revised Standard Version, Ecclesiastes 7, "A Disillusioned View of Life") and in study notes (see The Voice, Isaiah 60:19).
2. James A. Swanson, *Dictionary of Biblical Languages with Semantic Domains: Hebrew (Old Testament),* Logos ed. (Bellingham, WA: Faithlife, 1997), s.v. "שֶׁקֶר (šĕ·qěr)."
3. Edward W. Goodrick and John R. Kohlenberger III, *The NIV Exhaustive Concordance* (Grand Rapids, MI: Zondervan, 1990), 1647.
4. Swanson, *Dictionary of Biblical Languages,* s.v. "חָתַת (hā-ṯǎṯ)."
5. Swanson, s.v. "בָּעַר (bā-'ǎr)."
6. Goodrick and Kohlenberger, *NIV Exhaustive Concordance.*
7. Swanson, *Dictionary of Biblical Languages,* s.v. "בּוֹשׁ (bôš)."

APPENDIX C: A BRIEF ETYMOLOGY OF DISILLUSIONMENT

1. *Oxford English Dictionary Online,* s.v. "disillusion *(noun),*" accessed August 7, 2022, https://www.oed.com/view/Entry/54534.
2. Elizabeth Barrett Browning, *Casa Guidi Windows: A Poem (1851)* (1851; repr., Kessinger Legacy Reprints, Whitefish, MT: Kessinger, 2010), vi–vii.
3. "A Day in Old Rome," *The Leisure Hour,* no. 254, November 6, 1856; *Oxford English Dictionary Online,* s.v. "disillusionment *(noun),*" accessed August 7, 2022, https://www.oed.com/view/Entry/54538.

APPENDIX D: A COMMENTARY ON RELATED TERMS AND CONCEPTS

1. As the bibliography confirms, many more scholars were consulted than are listed in the table. The reason for this is that not all scholars offered further contributions to the subject, but rather were summarizing or commenting upon the offerings of other scholars already listed.
2. Genesis 15:12.
3. The full quote reads, "Guide us to that topmost height of mystic lore which exceedeth light and more than exceedeth knowledge, where the simple, absolute, and unchangeable mysteries of heavenly Truth lie hidden in the dazzling obscurity of the secret Silence, outshining all brilliance with the intensity of their darkness, and surcharging our blinded intellects with the utterly impalpable and invisible fairness of glories which exceed all beauty!" Pseudo-Dionysius, *Dionysius the Areopagite,* "Mystical Theology," 1.192.
4. Evelyn Underhill, ed., *The Cloud of Unknowing: The Classic of Medieval Mysticism* (Mineola, NY: Dover Publications, 2003), loc. 507, Kindle.
5. Gerald G. May, *The Dark Night of the Soul: A Psychiatrist Explores the Connection between Darkness and Spiritual Growth* (San Francisco: HarperSanFrancisco, 2005), 75.
6. May, 47.
7. James S. Reitman, "God's 'Eye' for the *Imago Dei*: Wise Advocacy amid Disillusionment in Job and Ecclesiastes," *Trinity Journal* 31, no. 1 (March 1, 2010): 121.

8. Reitman, "God's 'Eye.'"

9. Reitman, "God's 'Eye.'"

10. Reitman, "God's 'Eye,'" 118. Reitman adds, "As with Job, a growing nihilism culminates in utter disillusionment at the pivot of the argument with the rhetorical question 'Who knows what is good for man . . . ?' (6:12a). This leads Qoheleth to turn to *wisdom* as the only viable means of finding any meaning in life (7:1-14)."

11. Reitman, "God's 'Eye.'"

12. Jerome T. Walsh, "Despair as a Theological Virtue in the Spirituality of Ecclesiastes," *Biblical Theology Bulletin* 12, no. 2 (April 1982): 48.

13. Simon D. Podmore, "Lazarus and the Sickness unto Death: An Allegory of Despair," *Religion and the Arts* 15, no. 4 (January 1, 2011): 491.

14. Philip Yancey, *Disappointment with God: Three Questions No One Asks Aloud* (Grand Rapids, MI: Zondervan, 1988), 165.

15. Diane Jacobson, "Job as a Theologian of the Cross," *Word and World* 31, no. 4 (September 1, 2011): 375.

16. Jacobson, "Job as a Theologian," 379. On the phrase "crushed theologians," Jacobson notes: "This marvelous phrase comes from Fred Reisz in an unpublished presentation at a conference of teaching theologians of the ELCA."

17. Jacobson, "Job as a Theologian," 376.

18. Jacobson, "Job as a Theologian," 379.

19. Peter J. Morden, "C. H. Spurgeon and Suffering," *Evangelical Review of Theology* 35, no. 4 (October 1, 2011): 320.

20. Charles H. Spurgeon, "The Pitifulness of the Lord the Comfort of the Afflicted," sermon, Metropolitan Tabernacle, Newington, June 14, 1885, no. 1845.

21. Morden, "C. H. Spurgeon and Suffering," 319.

22. Yancey, *Disappointment with God*, 232.

23. Sigmund Freud, "Mourning and Melancholia," in *The Standard Edition of the Complete Psychological Works of Sigmund Freud*, ed. James Strachey, vol. 14 (London: Hogarth Press, 1957).

24. Freud is well-known for his thoughts on the mother-infant relationship: specifically, the infantile disappointment of transition from oneness with the mother in the womb to separateness at birth and breast. According to Freud and many who followed him, this unavoidable separation and the subsequent experiences of de-idealization affect and shape the developing self.

25. Peter Homans, *The Ability to Mourn: Disillusionment and the Social Origins of Psychoanalysis* (Chicago: University of Chicago Press, 1989), 4.

26. Homans, *Ability to Mourn*, 211–12.

27. Merton states, "The study of Nature in a 'convincing, scientific way' furthers a full appreciation of the Creator's power, so that the natural scientist must needs be better equipped than the casual observer to glorify Him. In this direct fashion, religion sanctioned science and raised the social estimation of those who pursued scientific investigation." Robert K. Merton, *Science, Technology and Society in Seventeenth Century England* (New York: H. Fertig, 1970), 71–72. Previously published as "Science, Technology and Society in Seventeenth Century England," in *Osiris* 4 (1938): 360–632.

28. Merton, *Science, Technology and Society*, 66–67.
29. Homans, *Ability to Mourn*, 213–14.
30. Homans, 9.
31. Reitman, "God's 'Eye,'" 122.
32. Julian Norris Hartt, "The Significance of Despair in Contemporary Theology," *Theology Today* 13, no. 1 (April 1, 1956): 57.
33. Hartt, "Significance of Despair," 53.
34. Hartt, 53.
35. As Hartt illustrates, "Egypt's pyramids celebrate dramatically the scientific, artistic and political accomplishments of that world; but they are also a gesture of despair, they are tombs in the land of the living; and they are then at one and the same time acts of defiance and confessions of despair." Hartt, "Significance of Despair," 54.
36. Hartt, "Significance of Despair," 54.
37. Béla Vassady, "A Theology of Hope for the Philosophy of Despair," *Theology Today* 5, no. 2 (July 1, 1948): 162.
38. Vassady, "Theology of Hope," 163.
39. David R. Blumenthal, "Despair and Hope Late in Post-Shoah Life," originally published in *Bridges: An Interdisciplinary Journal of Theology, Philosophy, History, and Science* 6, nos. 3/4 (1999), DavidBlumenthal.org, http://davidblumenthal .org/DespairHope.html.
40. Blumenthal, "Despair and Hope."
41. Blumenthal, "Despair and Hope."
42. Søren Kierkegaard, *Fear and Trembling and The Sickness unto Death*, trans. Walter Lowrie (Princeton, NJ: Princeton University Press, 2013), 348.
43. Podmore interestingly points out that "in Kierkegaard's Danish, as well as the German of Luther and Holbein, the etymological root of 'despair' (Dan. *Fortvivlelse*; Ger. *Verzweifeln*) is in 'doubt' (Dan. *tvivl*; Ger. *zweifel*), while the prefixes denote intensification [*for-/ver-*]; as such, *Fortvivlelse* and *Verzweifeln* both literally mean 'intensified doubt.'" Kierkegaard's personal despair seems to, at least in part, be related to doubt that he could be truly forgiven. Podmore, "Lazarus," 489.
44. Simon D. Podmore, "Kierkegaard as Physician of the Soul: On Self-Forgiveness and Despair," *Journal of Psychology and Theology* 37, no. 3 (September 1, 2009): 178.
45. Podmore, 181.
46. Podmore, 181.
47. Thomas Merton, *No Man Is an Island* (New York: Harcourt, 1983), 237–38.
48. Yancey, *Disappointment with God*, 64.
49. Douglas John Hall, *God and Human Suffering: An Exercise in the Theology of the Cross* (Minneapolis: Augsburg, 1986), 156.
50. Yancey, *Disappointment with God*, 234.
51. Yancey, 193–94.
52. C. S. Lewis, *The Screwtape Letters: With Screwtape Proposes a Toast*, rev. ed. (New York: Collier Books, 1982), 13–14.

53. In making this claim, I acknowledge the dissenting view of James Davison Hunter, who asserts that cultures change when an idea or belief is embraced and championed by elite and scholars near the "center" of cultural power who (1) forge the idea into an "intellectual framework," (2) network intentionally with one another, (3) communicate with (and are consequently supported by) institutional influencers, and (4) write and distribute their writings in such a way that the concepts reach the masses. See James Davison Hunter, *To Change the World: The Irony, Tragedy, and Possibility of Christianity in the Late Modern World* (New York: Oxford University Press, 2010), 75–96. However, if we were to ask the American church to identify what influences have shaped their working theology of suffering, I believe that popular songs, paperback books, and downloadable podcasts would top the list of felt influences. While it may be quite true that culture only changes by the movement of elites and scholars, the daily life of Jesus-followers is deeply affected by popular media.

Bibliography

Aglen, Anthony Stocker. "Psalms." In *A Bible Commentary for English Readers*, edited by Charles John Ellicott. London: Cassell, 1905. Ellicott's Commentary for English Readers. Psalm 42. Bible Hub. https://biblehub.com/commentaries/ellicott/psalms /42.htm.

Allender, Dan B., and Tremper Longman III. *The Cry of the Soul: How Our Emotions Reveal Our Deepest Questions about God.* Colorado Springs: NavPress, 1994.

Augustine of Hippo. *Expositions on the Book of Psalms.* Vol. 1. Oxford, 1847.

Averbeck, Richard E. "The Human Spirit in Spiritual Formation." Paper presented at the Evangelical Theological Society International Annual Meeting, San Antonio, TX, November 2004.

Bass, Diana Butler. *A People's History of Christianity: The Other Side of the Story.* New York: HarperOne, 2010. Kindle.

Berthold-Bond, Daniel. "Lunar Musings? An Investigation of Hegel's and Kierkegaard's Portraits of Despair." *Religious Studies* 34, no. 1 (March 1998): 33–59.

Blumenthal, David R. "Despair and Hope in Post-Shoah Jewish Life." Originally published in *Bridges: An Interdisciplinary Journal of Theology, Philosophy, History, and Science* 6, nos. 3/4 (1999). DavidBlumental.org. http://davidblumenthal .org/DespairHope.html.

Boa, Kenneth. *Conformed to His Image: Biblical and Practical Approaches to Spiritual Formation.* Grand Rapids, MI: Zondervan, 2001.

Bonhoeffer, Dietrich. *The Cost of Discipleship.* New York: Touchstone, 1995.

Browning, Elizabeth Barrett. *Casa Guidi Windows: A Poem (1851).* Kessinger Legacy Reprints. Whitefish, MT: Kessinger, 2010.

Carrigan, Henry L., Jr., ed. *The Wisdom of the Desert Fathers and Mothers.* Paraclete Essentials. Brewster, MA: Paraclete Press, 2010.

Chambers, Oswald. *Baffled to Fight Better: Job and the Problem of Suffering.* Grand Rapids, MI: Discovery House, 1990.

———. *Leagues of Light: Diary of Oswald Chambers 1915–1917.* Louisville, KY: Operation Appreciation Ministries, 1984.

———. *My Utmost for His Highest.* Uhrichsville, OH: Barbour, 1991.

Cho, John Chongnahm. "Adam's Fall and God's Grace: Wesley's Theological Anthropology." In *Holiness as a Root of Morality*, edited by John S. Park, 3–16. Lewiston, NY: Edwin Mellen Press, 2006.

Chole, Alicia Britt. *Anonymous: Jesus' Hidden Years . . . and Yours*. Franklin, TN: Integrity, 2006.

———. *Finding an Unseen God: Reflections of a Former Atheist*. Bloomington, MN: Bethany House, 2008.

———. *40 Days of Decrease: A Different Kind of Hunger, a Different Kind of Fast*. Nashville: W Publishing Group, an imprint of Thomas Nelson, 2015.

———. *The Sacred Slow: A Holy Departure from Fast Faith*. Nashville: Thomas Nelson, 2017.

———. *Sitting in God's Sunshine, Resting in His Love*. Nashville: JCountryman, 2005.

Christensen, Philip H. "The Fall of Adam." *Anglican Theological Review* 92, no. 4 (September 1, 2010): 830.

Christian Classics Ethereal Library. https://www.ccel.org/.

Coe, John H. "Musings on the Dark Night of the Soul: Insights from St. John of the Cross on a Developmental Spirituality." *Journal of Psychology and Theology* 28, no. 4 (2000): 293–307.

———. "Resisting the Temptation of Moral Formation: Opening to Spiritual Formation in the Cross and the Spirit." *Journal of Spiritual Formation and Soul Care* 1, no. 1 (March 1, 2008): 54–78.

Coe, John H., and Todd W. Hall. *Psychology in the Spirit: Contours of a Transformational Psychology*. Downers Grove, IL: IVP Academic, 2010.

Coombs, Marie Theresa, and Francis Kelly Nemeck. *The Spiritual Journey: Critical Thresholds and Stages of Adult Spiritual Genesis*. Collegeville, MN: Liturgical Press, 1991.

"A Day in Old Rome." *The Leisure Hour*, no. 254, November 6, 1856.

Dillard, Annie. *Teaching a Stone to Talk: Expeditions and Encounters*. New York: HarperPerennial, 1992.

Early Christian Writings. http://earlychristianwritings.com/.

Emmert, Kevin. "Resting in the Work of God: The Forgotten Spiritual Discipline." *Christianity Today* 56, no. 3 (March 1, 2012): 36–37.

Eusebius. *Church History*. Book 5. New Advent. https://www.newadvent.org/fathers/250105.htm.

Faricy, Robert. "Teilhard de Chardin's Spirituality of the Cross." *Horizons* 3, no. 1 (March 1, 1976): 1–15.

Ferguson, Everett. *Early Christians Speak: Faith and Life in the First Three Centuries*. Vol. 2. 3rd ed. Abilene, TX: ACU Press, 2002.

———, ed. *Inheriting Wisdom: Readings for Today from Ancient Christian Writers*. Peabody, MA: Hendrickson, 2004.

Finnie, Kellsye M. *William Carey: By Trade a Cobbler*. Eastbourne, England: Kingsway, 1986.

Foster, Richard J. *Streams of Living Water: Celebrating the Great Traditions of Christian Faith*. New York: HarperCollins, 2001.

Foster, Richard J., and James Bryan Smith, eds. *Devotional Classics: Selected Readings for Individuals and Groups*. San Francisco: HarperSanFrancisco, 1993.

Freud, Sigmund. "Mourning and Melancholia." In *The Standard Edition of the Complete Psychological Works of Sigmund Freud*. Edited by James Strachey. Vol. 14. London: Hogarth Press, 1957.

Frey, Robert Seitz, ed. "Despair and Hope Late in the Twentieth Century." *Bridges: An Interdisciplinary Journal of Theology, Philosophy, History, and Science* 6 (Fall/Winter 1999): 115–218.

Friedman, Edwin H. *Generation to Generation: Family Process in Church and Synagogue*. New York: Guilford, 2011.

Godin, Seth. *Tribes: We Need You to Lead Us*. New York: Portfolio, 2008.

Goodrick, Edward W., and John R. Kohlenberger III. *The NIV Exhaustive Concordance*. Grand Rapids, MI: Zondervan, 1990.

Graham, Billy. *Nearing Home: Life, Faith, and Finishing Well*. Nashville: Thomas Nelson, 2011.

Grassley, Edward B. "The Role of Suffering in the Development of Spiritual Maturity." DMin diss., Gordon-Conwell Theological Seminary, 2000.

Gusmer, Charles W. "The Purpose of the Scrutinies: An Insight from the Ignatian Exercises." *Worship* 65, no. 2 (March 1, 1991): 125–32.

Guyon, Jeanne. *Jeanne Guyon: An Autobiography*. New Kensington, PA: Whitaker House, 1997.

Hall, Douglas John. *God and Human Suffering: An Exercise in the Theology of the Cross*. Minneapolis: Augsburg, 1986.

Hartt, Julian Norris. "Significance of Despair in Contemporary Theology." *Theology Today* 13, no. 1 (April 1, 1956): 45–62.

Hegel, Georg Wilhelm Friedrich. *Phenomenology of Spirit*. Translated by Arnold V. Miller. Foreword by J. N. Findlay. Oxford, England: Clarendon Press, 1977.

Hendry, Erica R. "7 Epic Fails Brought to You by the Genius Mind of Thomas Edison." *Smithsonian*, November 20, 2013. https://www.smithsonianmag.com/innovation/7 -epic-fails-brought-to-you-by-the-genius-mind-of-thomas-edison-180947786/.

Hinrichs, Scott W. "Perspectives on Suffering: Exploring the Why Questions." DMin diss., Bethel Theological Seminary, 2002.

Holmes, Urban T., III. *A History of Christian Spirituality: An Analytical Introduction*. Harrisburg, PA: Morehouse, 2002.

Homans, Peter. *The Ability to Mourn: Disillusionment and the Social Origins of Psychoanalysis*. Chicago: University of Chicago Press, 1989.

Houston, James M. "The Future of Spiritual Formation." *Journal of Spiritual Formation and Soul Care* 4, no. 2 (September 1, 2011): 131–39.

Howard, Evan. "Three Temptations of Spiritual Formation." *Christianity Today*, December 9, 2002. https://www.christianitytoday.com/ct/2002/december9/4.46.html.

Hunter, James Davison. *To Change the World: The Irony, Tragedy, and Possibility of Christianity in the Late Modern World*. New York: Oxford University Press, 2010.

Irvin, Dale T., and Scott W. Sunquist. *History of the World Christian Movement: Earliest Christianity to 1453*. Maryknoll, NY: Orbis Books, 2001.

Jacobson, Diane L. "God's Natural Order: Genesis or Job?" In *"And God Saw That It Was Good": Essays on Creation and God in Honor of Terence E. Fretheim*, edited by Frederick J. Gaiser and Mark A. Throntveit, 49–56. *Word and World* Supplement Series 5. Saint Paul, MN: *Word and World*, Luther Seminary, 2006.

———. "Job as a Theologian of the Cross." *Word and World* 31, no. 4 (Fall 2011): 374–80.

Jenkins, Jerry B. *Hymns for Personal Devotions*. Chicago: Moody, 1989.

John of the Cross. *Dark Night of the Soul*. 3rd ed. Translated and edited by E. Allison Peers. New York: Image Books, 1959. Christian Classics Ethereal Library. https://ccel.org/ccel/john_cross/dark_night/dark_night.

———. *The Collected Works of St. John of the Cross*. Rev. ed. Translated by Kieran Kavanaugh and Otilio Rodriguez. Washington, DC: ICS Publications, 1991.

Kalantzis, George. "From the Porch to the Cross: Ancient Christian Approaches to Spiritual Formation." In *Life in the Spirit: Spiritual Formation in Theological Perspective*, edited by Jeffrey P. Greenman and George Kalantzis, 63–81. Downers Grove, IL: IVP Academic, 2010.

Kelly, Thomas R. *A Testament of Devotion*. New York: HarperOne, 1996.

à Kempis, Thomas. *The Imitation of Christ*. Rev. ed. New York: Grosset and Dunlap, 1926.

Kierkegaard, Søren. *Fear and Trembling and The Sickness unto Death*. Translated by Walter Lowrie. Princeton, NJ: Princeton University, 1974.

———. *The Sickness unto Death: A Christian Psychological Exposition for Upbuilding and Awakening*. Vol. 19, Kierkegaard's Writings. Edited and translated by Howard V. Hong and Edna H. Hong. Princeton pbk., with corrections. Princeton, NJ: Princeton University Press, 1983.

———. *Søren Kierkegaard: The Last Years, Journals 1853–1855*. Edited and translated by Ronald Gregor Smith. London: Lowe and Brydone, 1985.

Kirkpatrick, Alexander Francis. *Psalms: Books II & III*. Cambridge Bible for Schools and Colleges, edited by J. J. S. Perowne. Cambridge: Cambridge University Press, 1904. Psalm 42. Bible Hub. https://biblehub.com/commentaries/cambridge/psalms/42.htm.

Lambert, D. W. *Oswald Chambers: An Unbribed Soul*. 1983. Reprint, Fort Washington, PA: Christian Literature Crusade, 1989.

Lawrence, Brother, and Frank Laubach. *Practicing His Presence*. The Library of Spiritual Classics, Vol. 1. Jacksonville, FL: Christian Books, 1988.

Lewis, C. S. *A Grief Observed*. San Francisco: HarperSanFrancisco, 2001.

———. *Prince Caspian*. London: Geoffrey Bles, 1951. Reprint, New York: HarperCollins, 2005.

———. *The Screwtape Letters: With Screwtape Proposes a Toast*. Rev. ed. New York: Collier Books, 1982.

———. *The World's Last Night, and Other Essays*. (New York: Harcourt Brace, 1952; repr., San Francisco: HarperOne, 2017.

Lindberg, Carter. *The European Reformations*. 2nd ed. Malden, MA: Wiley-Blackwell, 2010.

MacDonald, George. *Diary of an Old Soul: 366 Writings for Devotional Reflection.* Minneapolis, MN: Augsburg Books, 1994.

Mandela, Nelson. *Long Walk to Freedom: The Autobiography of Nelson Mandela.* New York: Little, Brown, 1995.

May, Gerald G. *The Dark Night of the Soul: A Psychiatrist Explores the Connection between Darkness and Spiritual Growth.* 2003. Reprint, San Francisco: HarperSanFrancisco, 2005.

McFarland, Ian A. *In Adam's Fall: A Meditation on the Christian Doctrine of Original Sin.* Malden, MA: Wiley-Blackwell, 2010.

Mennekes, Friedhelm. "On the Spirituality of Questioning: James Lee Byars's *The White Mass* (1995) at the Kunst-Station Sankt Peter Cologne." *Religion and the Arts* 13, no. 3 (July 2009): 358–75.

Menzies, Allan, ed. *The Writings of the Fathers down to AD 325.* Vol. 3, *Latin Christianity: Its Founder, Tertullian.* Grand Rapids, MI: Eerdmans, 2009. Christian Classics Ethereal Library. https://www.ccel.org/ccel/schaff/anf03.i.html.

Merton, Robert K. *Science, Technology and Society in Seventeenth Century England.* New York: H. Fertig, 1970. Originally published in *Osiris* 4 (1938): 360–632.

Merton, Thomas. *No Man Is an Island.* Harvest/HBJ ed. New York: Harcourt, 1983.

———. *The Wisdom of the Desert.* New York: New Directions, 1970.

Moore, Chandler, Chris Brown, Naomi Rain, and Steven Furtick. "Jireh." Track 2, *Old Church Basement.* Elevation Worship/Maverick City Music. Released as a single March 26, 2021.

Morden, Peter J. "C. H. Spurgeon and Suffering." *Evangelical Review of Theology* 35, no. 4 (October 1, 2011): 306–25.

Norris, Kathleen. *The Cloister Walk.* New York: Riverhead Books, 1996.

Nouwen, Henri J. M. *In the Name of Jesus: Reflections on Christian Leadership with Study Guide for Groups and Individuals.* New York: Crossroad, 2002.

———. *Making All Things New: An Invitation to the Spiritual Life.* San Francisco: Harper and Row, 1981.

———. *The Way of the Heart: Connecting with God through Prayer, Wisdom, and Silence.* New York: Ballantine Books, 2003.

———. *The Wounded Healer: Ministry in Contemporary Society.* London: Darton Longman and Todd, 1994.

Nystrom, Martin J. "As the Deer." Universal Music/Brentwood-Benson Publishing, 1984.

Olson, Roger E. *The Story of Christian Theology: Twenty Centuries of Tradition and Reform.* Downers Grove, IL: IVP Academic, 1999.

Osbeck, Kenneth W. *101 Hymn Stories: The Inspiring True Stories behind 101 Favorite Hymns.* Grand Rapids, MI: Kregel, 2012.

Peterson, Eugene H. "Transparent Lives." *Christian Century*, November 29, 2003. https://www.christiancentury.org/article/2003-11/transparent-lives.

Phillips, Rachael. *Well with My Soul: Four Dramatic Stories of Great Hymn Writers.* Uhrichsville, OH: Barbour, 2003.

Podmore, Simon D. "Kierkegaard as Physician of the Soul: On Self-Forgiveness and Despair." *Journal of Psychology and Theology* 37, no. 3 (September 1, 2009): 174–85.

———. "Lazarus and the Sickness unto Death: An Allegory of Despair." *Religion and the Arts* 15, no. 4 (January 1, 2011): 486–519.

Pseudo-Dionysius. *Dionysius the Areopagite: On the Divine Names and the Mystical Theology.* Translated by C. E. Rolt. London: SPCK, 1920. Reprint, Whitefish, MT: Kessinger, 1992.

Reading, Anthony. *Hope and Despair: How Perceptions of the Future Shape Human Behavior.* Baltimore, MD: Johns Hopkins University Press, 2004.

Reitman, James S. "God's 'Eye' for the *Imago Dei*: Wise Advocacy amid Disillusionment in Job and Ecclesiastes." *Trinity Journal* 31, no. 1 (March 1, 2010): 115–34.

Robertson, Katharine. "Original Sin or Original Blessing?: How the Doctrine of Original Sin Paints a Distorted Picture of God and Human Nature, and the Effect This Has on Spiritual Formation." DMin diss., George Fox Evangelical Seminary, 2010.

Rusten, E. Michael, and Sharon O. Rusten. *The One Year Book of Christian History.* Carol Stream, IL: Tyndale, 2003.

The Sayings of the Desert Fathers: The Alphabetical Collection. Translated by Benedicta Ward. Rev. ed. Collegeville, MN: Cistercian Publications, 2006.

Schaff, Philip, ed. *Nicene and Post-Nicene Fathers.* Series 1, vol. 9, *Early Church Fathers.* Enhanced version. Grand Rapids, MI: Christian Classics Ethereal Library, 2009. Kindle.

Scholtes, Peter. "They'll Know We Are Christians by Our Love." 1966. F.E.L. Publications, assigned to The Lorenz Corp., 1991.

Scorgie, Glen G., Simon Chan, Gordon T. Smith, and James D. Smith III, eds. *Dictionary of Christian Spirituality.* Grand Rapids, MI: Zondervan, 2011.

Serra, Dominic E. "New Observations about the Scrutinies of the Elect in Early Roman Practice." *Worship* 80, no. 6 (November 1, 2006): 511–27.

Sewall, Richard B. *The Life of Emily Dickinson.* 2 vols. Cambridge, MA: Harvard University Press, 1994.

Sheldrake, Philip. *A Brief History of Spirituality.* Malden, MA: Wiley-Blackwell, 2007.

Shults, F. LeRon, and Steven J. Sandage. *Transforming Spirituality: Integrating Theology and Psychology.* Grand Rapids, MI: Baker Academic, 2006.

Smedes, Lewis B. *Shame and Grace: Healing the Shame We Don't Deserve.* San Francisco: HarperSanFrancisco, 1993.

Spafford Vester, Bertha. *Our Jerusalem: An American Family in the Holy City, 1881–1949.* LaVergne, TN: Ramsay Press, 2007.

Spitz, Elie Kaplan, with Erica Shapiro Taylor. *Healing from Despair: Choosing Wholeness in a Broken World.* Woodstock, VT: Jewish Lights, 2008.

Spurgeon, C. H. *The Autobiography of Charles H. Spurgeon: Compiled from His Diary, Letters, and Records by His Wife and His Private Secretary.* Vol. 2. Chicago: Fleming H. Revell, 1899.

———. "A Question for a Questioner." Sermon. Metropolitan Tabernacle, Newington, May 31, 1885. No. 1843.

———. "Deep Calleth unto Deep." Sermon. Metropolitan Tabernacle, Newington, April 11, 1869. No. 865. The Spurgeon Center for Biblical Preaching at Midwestern Seminary. https://www.spurgeon.org/resource-library/sermons/deep-calleth-unto-deep/#flipbook/.

———. "The Pitifulness of the Lord the Comfort of the Afflicted." Sermon. Metropolitan Tabernacle, Newington, June 14, 1885. No. 1845.

———. "3 June: Philippians 2:8." In *Evening by Evening*. London: Passmore and Alabaster, 1868.

———. *The Saint and His Saviour: or, The Progress of the Soul in the Knowledge of Jesus.* 1857. Reprint, London: Hodder and Stoughton, 1889.

Steinke, Peter L. *How Your Church Family Works: Understanding Congregations as Emotional Systems* (Herndon, VA: Alban Institute, 2006).

Stevens, Richard G. "We Don't Need More Sleep. We Just Need More Darkness." *Washington Post*, October 27, 2015. https://www.washingtonpost.com/posteverything/wp/2015/10/27/we-dont-need-more-sleep-we-just-need-more-darkness/.

Swanson, James A. *Dictionary of Biblical Languages with Semantic Domains: Hebrew (Old Testament)*. Logos ed. Bellingham, WA: Faithlife, 1997.

Sweet, Leonard. *I Am a Follower: The Way, Truth, and Life of Following Jesus*. Nashville: Thomas Nelson, 2012.

———. *The Well-Played Life: Why Pleasing God Doesn't Have to Be Such Hard Work.* Carol Stream, IL: Tyndale Momentum, 2014.

Sweet, Leonard, and Frank Viola. *Jesus Manifesto: Restoring the Supremacy and Sovereignty of Jesus Christ*. Nashville: Thomas Nelson, 2010. Kindle.

Taft, Robert F. "Lent: A Meditation." *Worship* 57, no. 2 (March 1, 1983): 123–25.

Teresa of Ávila. *Interior Castle*. Translated by E. Allison Peers. Radford, VA: Wilder Publications, 2008.

Thompson, Marianne Meye. "Turning and Returning to God: Reflections on the Lectionary Texts for Lent." *Interpretation* 64, no. 1 (January 1, 2010): 5–17.

Troxel, Ronald L., Kelvin G. Friebel, and Dennis R. Magary, eds. *Seeking out the Wisdom of the Ancients: Essays Offered to Honor Michael V. Fox on the Occasion of His Sixty-Fifth Birthday*. Winona Lake, IN: Eisenbrauns, 2005.

Turgenev, Ivan Sergeevich. *The Essential Turgenev*. Edited by Elizabeth Cheresh Allen. Evanston, IL: Northwestern University Press, 1994.

Tyson, John R., ed. *Invitation to Christian Spirituality: An Ecumenical Anthology*. New York: Oxford University Press, 1999.

Underhill, Evelyn, ed. *The Cloud of Unknowing: The Classic of Medieval Mysticism*. Mineola, NY: Dover Publication, 2003. Kindle.

Vassady, Béla. "A Theology of Hope for the Philosophy of Despair." *Theology Today* 5, no. 2 (July 1, 1948): 158–73.

Veith, Gene Edward, Jr. *Loving God with All Your Mind: Thinking as a Christian in the Postmodern World*. Rev. ed. Wheaton, IL: Crossway Books, 2003.

Votaw, Dave. "How to Be a Quaker in the Twenty-First Century." MA thesis, George Fox University, 1997.

Walsh, Jerome T. "Despair as a Theological Virtue in the Spirituality of Ecclesiastes." *Biblical Theology Bulletin* 12, no. 2 (April 1982): 46–49.

Wheatley, Margaret J. *Leadership and the New Science: Discovering Order in a Chaotic World.* 3rd ed. San Francisco: Berrett-Koehler, 2006. Kindle.

Williams, Rowan. *The Wound of Knowledge: Christian Spirituality from the New Testament to St. John of the Cross.* 2nd rev. ed. Cambridge, MA: Cowley Publications, 1991.

Williams, Stephen N. Review of *In Adam's Fall: A Meditation on the Christian Doctrine of Original Sin*, by Ian A. McFarland. *Evangelical Quarterly* 84, no. 2 (April 1, 2012): 185–88.

Woodbridge, John D., ed. *Ambassadors for Christ: Distinguished Representatives of the Message throughout the World.* Chicago: Moody, 1994.

Yancey, Philip. *Disappointment with God: Three Questions No One Asks Aloud.* Grand Rapids, MI: Zondervan, 1988.

About the Author

In person or in print, Dr. Alicia Britt Chole's voice cuts through fluff and summons souls to walk with God anew. As a speaker, leadership mentor, and award-winning writer, Alicia places words like an artist applying paint to a canvas. Nothing is wasted. Every word matters. Heads and hearts are equally engaged. A former atheist, Alicia's worldview was interrupted by Jesus as she began her university studies. Of that experience Alicia states, "I would have had to commit emotional and intellectual suicide to deny God's reality." Today, her raw faith and love for God's Word hold the attention of saints and skeptics alike. Alicia focuses on less than trendy topics like spiritual pain, the leader's soul, the potential of anonymous years, decrease as a discipline, and the abuse of authority. Business leaders, pastors, college students, and churches agree: Alicia is an unusually disarming combination of realism and hope, intellect and grace, humor and art. Alicia and Barry have been married for thirty years. Along with their three amazing children (all Choles through the miracle of adoption), they live in the country off of a dirt road in the Ozarks. Alicia holds a doctorate in leadership and spiritual formation from George Fox Evangelical Seminary and is the founding director and lead mentor of Leadership Investment Intensives, Inc., a nonprofit devoted to providing confidential and customized soul-care to leaders in the marketplace and church. Her favorite things include thunderstorms, honest questions, LOTR, and anything with jalapeños. In a culture obsessed with things new and countable, Alicia brings ancient truth to life.